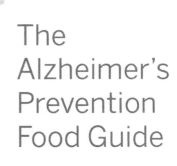

The
Alzheimer's
Prevention
Food Guide

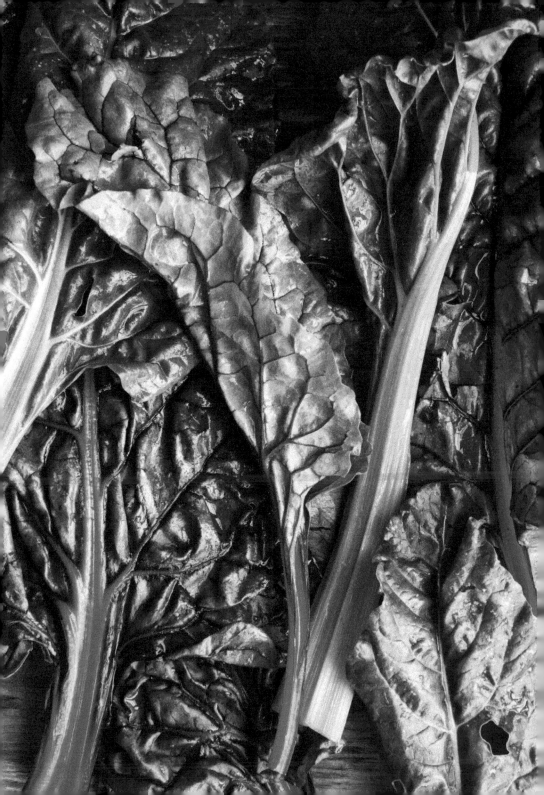

The
Alzheimer's
Prevention
Food Guide

{ A Quick Nutritional Reference to
Foods that Nourish and Protect the
Brain from Alzheimer's Disease

SUE STILLMAN LINJA, RDN, LD
SEANNE SAFAII-WAITE, PHD, RDN, LD

**ROCKRIDGE
PRESS**

Design by Debbie Berne

Cover photography: Toma Evsiukova/Stocksy; back cover: Pixel Stories/Stocksy; Joe Pallen; Interior photography: Sara Remington/Stocksy, p.ii; Pixel Stories/Stocksy, p.vi; Julien L Balmer/Stocksy, p.vii; Pixel Stories/Stocksy, p.xiv; DOBRÁNSKA RENÁTA/Stocksy, p.20; Ina Peters/Stocksy, p.38; Darren Muir/Stocksy, p.43; B.&.E.Dudzinski/Stockfood, p.53; etorres/Shutterstock, p.57; AnjelikaGr/Shutterstock, p.67; Alexey Kuzma/Stocksy, p.71; Oliver Wilde/Shutterstock, p.77; Zocky/Stocksy, p.87; Kema Food Culture/Stocksy, p.89; Jeff Wasserman/Stocksy, p.93; Silberkorn/Shutterstock, p.97; Veronika Studer/Stocksy, p.98; Toma Evsiukova/Stocksy, p.128; Sue Stillman Linja, p.176; University of Idaho p.176

ISBN: Print 978-1-62315-908-5 | eBook 978-1-62315-909-2

We dedicate this book to our beautiful mothers,
Sarah Schwartz and Gloria Schuch

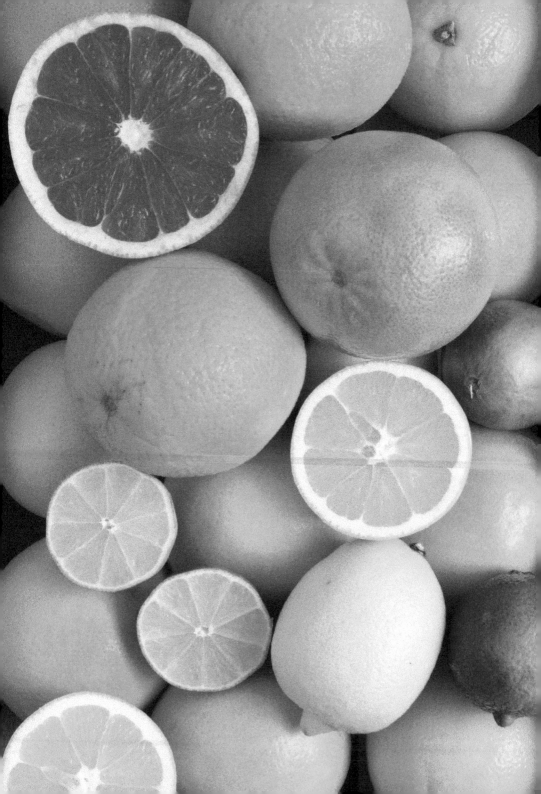

Contents

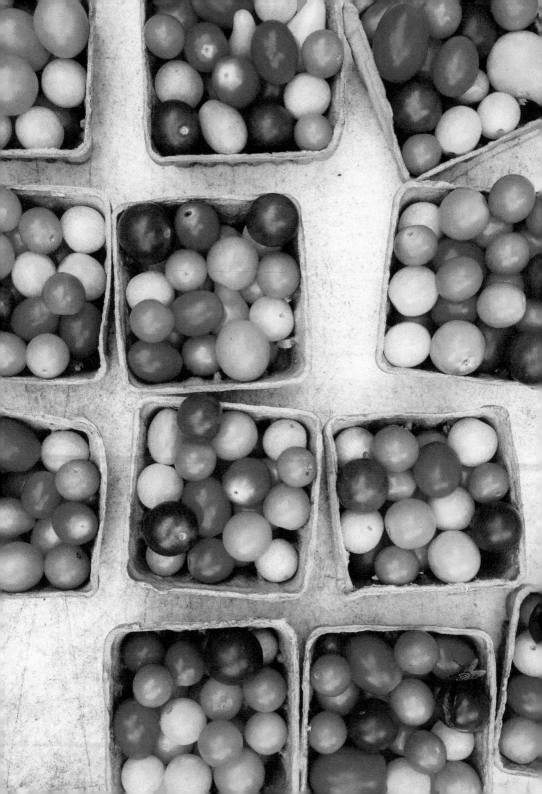

Introduction

Two registered dietitian nutritionists. Two daughters of Alzheimer's victims. Two heartfelt stories converge. We hope our voice on prevention will speak for those who no longer can, like our mothers, and will provide knowledge and guidance to others who may be trying to avoid this complex and debilitating disease.

Sue's Story

My mom felt she was put on this earth to feed her family and friends. My siblings and I called it "Italian food torture." Up at the crack of dawn to start the chicken stock, she'd then move on to making sourdough pancakes for six hungry kids. At midnight, she'd still be up, folding laundry or making homemade pasta. My mom rarely slept. Always with a smile on her face, she cooked and cleaned and loved and dreamed, but she rarely slept.

Did her lifestyle, including the lack of consistent sleep, contribute to the devastating disease that turned my sweet, smiling mom into someone I didn't recognize? Or could it have been the slow change from the Mediterranean-style diet of her childhood (which included lots of olive oil, vegetables, and very little meat) to a Western diet that satisfied my dad's desire for meat and rich foods?

Either way, my mom is no longer with us. Alzheimer's disease shattered her dreams and stole the life she knew. My mom died bearing no resemblance to her former self, except perhaps her beaming smile.

SeAnne's Story

I remember my father telling me one day that I needed to watch my mom closely because something wasn't right. "She keeps forgetting things," he said. "She left the stove on yesterday." I brushed this off as simple forgetfulness. After all, I too am forgetful at times.

We had no history of dementia or Alzheimer's disease in our family, so I really wasn't worried. Yet within a year I started noticing her inability to carry on deep conversations, her occasional blank looks, and her complaints of getting mixed up a lot.

One day my mom went out on her daily walk and wound up several neighborhoods away, exhausted, dehydrated, and lost. Similar occurrences took place after that. Eventually, we placed her in a memory care facility, where she still resides today. This once-athletic, happy, and loving woman had become agitated, angry, confused and, at times, catatonic. She is not yet gone, but I miss her.

Our experiences are personal, but unfortunately they are not unique to us. Alzheimer's disease statistics in the United States are staggering: According to the Alzheimer's Association, about 5.4 million Americans are living with the disease, and this number is on the rise. Today, one in three seniors dies with Alzheimer's or dementia, and although deaths from other major diseases have decreased significantly in the last decade, Alzheimer's deaths have increased by 71 percent. Given that there is not a cure for Alzheimer's, medical communities are looking to prevention to slow down these alarming increases. Exercise, diet, and brain activities all show great preventive promise. In light of our interests and expertise, this book dives exclusively into the food, nutrition, and diet component. Although diet is important for all types of dementia, this guide focuses on the prevention of Alzheimer's disease.

Food as medicine has been an important doctrine in countries and cultures around the globe for centuries. A nutritious diet can not only help prevent chronic disease, but is often used as a treatment for disease. We know, too, that unhealthy diets can have devastating effects on the human body. They can exponentially shorten lives and are the root cause of many common diseases.

This is the first and only detailed food guide written to assist you with making brain-healthy dietary alterations and incorporating mind-nourishing foods into your diet—all without making drastic changes. This guide will modify the way you think about the foods you eat and give you ways to fortify your brain. You will learn

- why diet can protect against Alzheimer's disease.
- how healthy and unhealthy foods affect your brain.

- which foods—more than 100 of them—you can incorporate into your diet, and why they are beneficial.
- how easy it is to add brain-healthy foods to your daily meal plan.

As dietitians and researchers, we have spent a great deal of time investigating the links between diet and Alzheimer's disease. Cutting-edge research continues to explore the fascinating science behind nutrition and cognition, and further exploration will result in even more compelling dietary recommendations. For now, this guide can be used by those of you who are interested in promoting a healthy brain and preventing or delaying cognitive decline as you age. Please join us on our journey to marry nutrition science and optimism in the prevention of Alzheimer's disease.

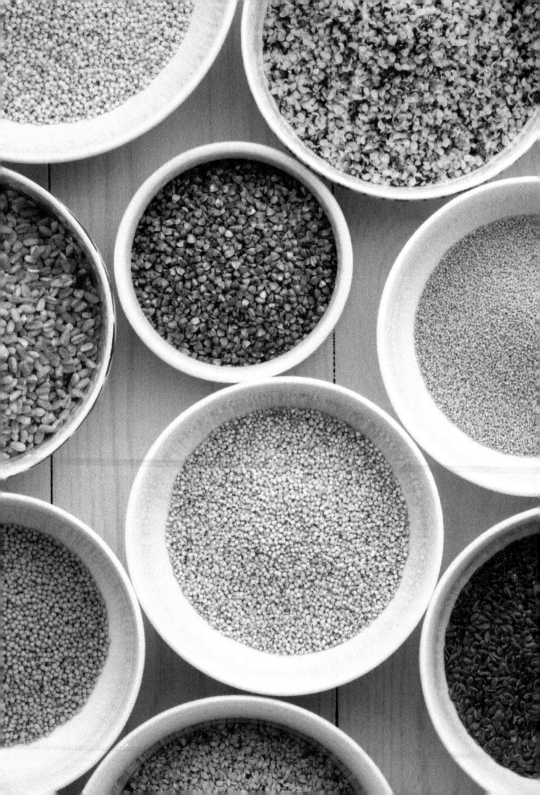

Chapter 1
The Alzheimer's–Diet Connection

Many experts, ourselves included, argue that the only way to reduce the risk of Alzheimer's disease is to adopt a healthy lifestyle by participating in regular exercise; staying mentally active; maintaining normal blood pressure, blood sugar, and blood fat levels; and eating plenty of brain-healthy foods. The connection between consumption of the current Western diet and the development of Alzheimer's is becoming more evident, and the research for making beneficial changes to one's diet is more compelling. While consuming a healthy diet is not a magic bullet to remove all risk of developing the disease or to reverse Alzheimer's, it does show promise for those with no current signs or symptoms of cognitive loss.

Alzheimer's Basics

The brain is the most complicated system in the body, connecting every organ and function necessary to live. The frontal and temporal lobes of the cerebrum and the limbic system house memory. In conjunction with the neurons and neurotransmitters, the brain's communication mechanism enables a healthy body to move, think, speak, and feel. A control center for the rest of the body, the brain is not easily understood or simply explained.

Your brain is always "on," whether you are awake or asleep. And since it is running, it needs the proper mix of nutrients all the time, day and night. To use an analogy, the brain is like an aircraft. While an aircraft can run on simple car gas, it needs specialized lubricants, fluids, and gasoline to work efficiently. Your brain is like the aircraft; it needs a variety of nutrients to function effectively. An airplane *can* run on car gasoline and your brain *can* function when you eat unhealthy foods. But in the long term, in either scenario, the wrong fuel can have serious negative effects, resulting in deterioration of the system.

If your brain lacks the nutrients it needs to complete its complicated functions, like the aircraft running on car fuel, it will falter.

Alzheimer's disease disrupts critical metabolic pathways in the brain. Researchers have found that the damage in the brain of someone with Alzheimer's begins about a decade before symptoms appear. As the disease progresses, leading to the outward symptoms of Alzheimer's, the brain starts to show deposits of proteins known as amyloid plaques and tau protein tangles. With the increase of these deposits, once-healthy neurons in the brain die. Brain tissue and function is damaged, and the brain shrinks significantly.

DEFINING
Alzheimer's and Dementia

Alzheimer's disease is a nonreversible brain disorder that develops slowly and progresses to the point of completely diminished short-term memory and total debilitation. Many people use the terms *dementia* and *Alzheimer's* interchangeably, but in fact they are not the same.

Dementia is the overarching term for the loss of brain function including reasoning, thinking, and recall.

Alzheimer's disease accounts for 60 to 80 percent of all dementia cases, according to the Alzheimer's Association. While there are many different types of dementia, Alzheimer's disease is by far the most common.

There are two diagnostic stages of Alzheimer's:

Mild cognitive impairment (MCI) due to Alzheimer's disease, where cognitive decline is greater than expected given a person's age and education but does not significantly interfere with everyday activities.

Dementia due to Alzheimer's disease, which is characterized by noticeable cognition symptoms that impair a person's ability to function in daily life.

There is also a preclinical stage, which a person can be in before symptoms such as memory loss develop. Due to the lack of symptoms, an individual cannot know if he or she is in a preclinical phase. Researchers are just beginning to study the preclinical brain thanks to individuals who volunteer to be research subjects. These people have no symptoms but suspect (for one reason or another) that they might be at risk of developing Alzheimer's.

The Rise in Alzheimer's

The Alzheimer's Association pegs Alzheimer's disease as the most under-recognized public health concern of the century. Today in the United States, one in nine people over the age of 65 has been diagnosed with Alzheimer's disease, and millions more cases remain undiagnosed. Scarier still, the death rate is increasing—Alzheimer's is officially the sixth leading cause of death in America, and the fifth leading cause of death in the elderly. Nearly one person each minute develops Alzheimer's, and by 2050 this is projected to be one every 33 seconds. The risk of developing the disease doubles every five years after the age of 65, and since Americans are living longer—many into their eighties and nineties—scientists predict that by midcentury 13.8 million people will be living with Alzheimer's.

Unlike with many other chronic diseases, the cause of Alzheimer's is not clear. Improved diagnostics have identified more cases; incidence increases with age, as expected, but what else is behind the staggering increase in this deadly disease? Later in this chapter, we explore potential connections between Alzheimer's and insulin, diabetes, and inflammation. Many experts are convinced poor lifestyle and diet are leading contributors to Alzheimer's, as they are for other chronic diseases such as heart disease and type 2 diabetes. Because we know that exercise and a healthy diet reduce the risk of inflammatory diseases such as diabetes, cardio-vascular disease, obesity, and cancer, it is also likely these lifestyle adjustments can reduce the risk of Alzheimer's through the same or similar mechanisms.

Who Is at Risk?

It is widely accepted that Alzheimer's disease is a complex and irreversible brain disorder that results from progressive brain cell death. It is also common knowledge that there are many risk factors associated with the disease. Although the multiple causal factors are complicated, having a basic appreciation of them can be empowering. Understanding the risk factors associated with Alzheimer's disease can help you be proactive and put together an individualized prevention plan. For simplicity, risk factors can be categorized as those that are unchangeable (age, race, gender and sex, brain injury, genetics, and family history) and changeable (diet, physical activity, sleep, tobacco use, education, exposure to general anesthesia, cognitive activity). While there are no certain characteristics to guarantee protection from Alzheimer's disease, it is helpful to understand more about some of the key risk factors.

Age

Age is rated as the greatest risk factor for developing Alzheimer's, but fortunately the disease is not a normal part of aging. Few young people are diagnosed with the disease—only 4 percent of the total population living with Alzheimer's is under age 65. The risk rises significantly with age: 81 percent of people with the disease are over 75 years of age, and one-third of elders over age 85 develop Alzheimer's. In addition, as the body ages, the body's decreased ability to repair its organs (including the brain) and the increased risk factors for cardiovascular disease also play a role in this disease.

Gender and Sex

The debate continues regarding Alzheimer's risk associated with the gender and sex of a person. About two-thirds of people living with Alzheimer's are women. Some research suggests the risk is higher for women due to biological or genetic variations (sex) or less access to education or occupational choices (gender) in the first half of the twentieth century. Men have a higher death rate from cardiovascular disease before the age of 65; therefore, men living into their later years may have a better cardiovascular risk profile and thus less risk of developing Alzheimer's. The best-known Alzheimer's disease genetic risk factor, the APOE-e4 gene, may have a stronger association among women than among men, possibly due to its connection to estrogen, which is more prevalent in women.

Cardiovascular Disease

Healthy heart, healthy brain. Cardiovascular factors, including heart disease, stroke, high blood pressure, and high cholesterol, cause damage to the heart or blood vessels and have been strongly linked to the development of Alzheimer's disease. Growing evidence suggests brain health is closely associated with the health of the heart and blood vessels. A healthy heart and healthy blood vessels help ensure the brain receives the oxygen and nutrients necessary to function normally.

People with high blood pressure and/or high blood cholesterol during midlife are more likely to develop Alzheimer's disease than those who are free from these conditions. The association between chronic inflammation, cardiovascular disease, and Alzheimer's will be discussed later in this chapter.

Diabetes

The link between Alzheimer's and diabetes is actively being investigated. Diabetes causes damage to blood vessels important for carrying nutrients and oxygen to the brain. Another link may be the complex way diabetes affects the ability of the brain to use sugar and respond to insulin. The insulin response to sugary Western diet meals (with resulting increases in dangerous beta-amyloid proteins in spinal fluids and a temporary decrease in cognitive abilities) is currently being studied at Wake Forest School of Medicine and by a neuropathologist-led research team at Brown University.

Many people with diabetes—especially type 2 diabetes—have changes in their brains characteristic of Alzheimer's disease. There are also correlations between type 2 diabetes and damaging protein deposits and brain tangles. Diabetic patients have a higher incidence of obesity and/or chronically high blood sugar levels, which may cause these brain changes. Older adults with diabetes have shown more brain shrinkage and a higher incidence of stroke than those without. Ultimately, people with type 2 diabetes have twice the risk of developing Alzheimer's disease. We anticipate that there will be further research investigating the relationship between Alzheimer's, insulin utilization, prediabetes, diabetes, and obesity.

Family History and Genetics

Alzheimer's risk related to family history and genetics is complicated. It is known that a person having a parent, sibling, or child with the disease increases the likelihood of him or her developing Alzheimer's—the risk goes up if more than one family member has the disease. Disorders with a familial link also often have a heredity association, and a lot of attention is being paid to the connection between the two.

Researchers have found Alzheimer's gene mutations in two categories: deterministic genes and risk genes. In people with early-onset Alzheimer's (ages 30 to 65), deterministic genes have been identified and are thought to be the direct cause of the disease. However, with late-onset Alzheimer's (after age 65), the genetic link is not as clear. There is no single gene mutation that consistently causes late-onset Alzheimer's.

The genetic links that do exist are risk genes, and while they increase the likelihood of developing Alzheimer's, they do not guarantee it. APOE-e4 is the risk gene with the greatest impact. If this gene is inherited from both parents, there is a higher likelihood of developing the brain disorder. It is estimated that 20 to 25 percent of all late-onset Alzheimer's is related to the APOE-e4 connection. APOE, though the best-known gene factor associated with Alzheimer's, is only one of many genes that contribute to the risk for developing late-onset Alzheimer's. Due to the complexity of the genetic link and the questionable association with Alzheimer's incidence, physicians discourage patients from getting genetic testing. It is important to remember that genetics alone do not dictate whether one does or does not develop Alzheimer's disease; the controllable risk factors are where energy should be focused.

Surprisingly, even though the United States is one of the top 10 wealthiest countries, it does not make the cut when it comes to longevity.

Do People Live Longest?

When we look at population health and longevity, we can rank the places in the world where people's life expectancy is the longest. For the most part, the more developed the economy, the longer the life expectancy—likely related to higher-quality health care and healthier diets. Surprisingly, even though the United States is one of the top 10 wealthiest countries, it does not make the cut when it comes to longevity. The average life expectancy in the United States is 78.7 years. These are the five countries with the longest average life expectancies:

1. Hong Kong (83.5 years)
2. Japan (83.1 years)
3. Spain (83.1 years)
4. Italy (82.9 years)
5. Switzerland (82.7 years)

Since the United States is a wealthy country with high-quality health care, could diet be the reason for increased Alzheimer's rates? The top five countries listed have diets composed primarily of whole foods, grains, fruits, vegetables, and fish. Residents of these countries consume foods with extremely high amounts of brain-healthy nutrients. Residents of Japan have a much lower rate of Alzheimer's than Americans; however, Japanese-Americans have higher rates than those living in Japan. This indicates diet, not genetics, may be the primary driver of Alzheimer's disease.

A Brief Overview of Nutrition and Brain Health

Our brains work hard around the clock. For that reason, the brain expends an enormous amount of energy and requires a constant supply of fuel and nutrients. There are three macronutrients—protein, carbohydrates, and fat—that are the main components of our diets and are essential for health. Too little or too much of these may result in poor health.

Macronutrients

Macronutrients provide the body with energy, and our bodies need these in the largest quantities. Macronutrients fall into three types: protein, carbohydrates, and fats.

Protein

Proteins are often referred to as the body's building blocks because they build and repair tissues. The amino acids that make up proteins are used for building DNA, cell membranes, hormones, receptors, and brain chemicals. Chemical messengers in the brain, called neurotransmitters, are made of amino acids.

The brain cannot function without protein. Older adults need to evenly distribute their protein intake throughout the day to maximize muscle health. The body's protein tank needs only 4 ounces of protein in one sitting (about 25 to 30 grams) to be filled; more than that and protein's muscle-building potential is squandered. Protein consumed above this threshold is stored primarily as fat. The average American eats very little protein for breakfast and often too much at the evening meal. Distributing protein intake throughout all three daily meals is important for maximizing the use of amino acids for brain health and may provide yet another tool for Alzheimer's prevention.

Carbohydrates

Carbohydrates are the body's and brain's primary source of energy. They break down into glucose during digestion. They are primarily plant based and make up the majority of calories in a meal. There are two types of carbohydrates: simple and complex.

> **Simple carbohydrates** are found in fruits, vegetables, and milk products as well as in sweeteners like sugar, honey, and syrup, and foods like desserts, pastries, candy, and soft drinks.
>
> **Complex carbohydrates** are found in breads, cereals, pasta, rice, beans, and starchy vegetables such as potatoes, squash, green peas, and corn.

It is advisable for most people to eat carbohydrates that contain higher amounts of fiber, often found in plant-based foods. Adding fiber to the diet helps prevent stomach and intestinal issues and can help reduce high blood sugar, which is increasingly linked to cognitive decline.

Fats

In addition to providing calories and satiety, fats are important for the absorption of vitamins and minerals. Here are the different categories of fats:

> **Polyunsaturated** fats include omega-3 fatty acids (fatty fish, walnuts, and some seeds like flax) and omega-6 fatty acids (corn, soybean, sesame oil; it's also used in products such as chips,

fast foods, candies, and pastries). Both types of fatty acids are needed and must be obtained from food since the body can't manufacture them.

Monounsaturated fats include canola, olive, peanut, and safflower oils; they are also found in avocados, peanut butter, and some nuts and seeds.

Saturated fats include palm and coconut oils and are also found in red meat, butter, and other solid fats. Meat, full-fat cheese, pizza, and desserts are common sources of saturated fats.

Trans fats are found in stick margarine and vegetable shortening. Trans fatty acids are often used in prepackaged foods, baked goods, and fried foods at some fast-food restaurants. Studies overwhelmingly support the avoidance of trans fats to promote optimal health.

About 60 percent of brain matter consists of fats. Specific fats are very important for brain health, while others can be detrimental. Excess intake of damaging fats like trans fats and saturated fats can increase your blood cholesterol levels and is linked to the development of Alzheimer's disease.

Micronutrients

Micronutrients are essential nutrients the body requires in the smallest quantities. They are made up of vitamins and minerals. They often have antioxidant properties, which can protect against damage to the cells of the body. A piece of metal left out in the elements for a long time starts to rust, or oxidize. A similar process happens inside the body. Antioxidants help protect against the chemical reaction of free radicals, to reduce their harmful effects.

Fatty Acids and Brain Health

Polyunsaturated fats (omega-3 and omega-6 fatty acids) are the most important fats for brain health.

- Omega-3 fatty acids have an anti-inflammatory effect.
- Omega-6 fatty acids cause inflammation or are pro-inflammatory.

We need to consume both types of fatty acids to create a balance and regulate inflammation. With an inflammatory response in the body, chemicals from white blood cells are released to protect the body from foreign substances, which is a good thing. But when inflammation becomes chronic, it promotes the development of a number of serious conditions such as cardiovascular disease, type 2 diabetes, and Alzheimer's disease. Our modern diet is too high in omega-6 fats and too low in omega-3s (up to 20 times more omega-6), increasing the risk of inflammatory diseases.

Dietary consumption of omega-3 fatty acids and its effect on the brain is one of the best-studied interactions between food and brain evolution. Docosahexaenoic acid (DHA) is a vital and abundant omega-3 fatty acid in brain cells; however, the human body is not efficient at synthesizing DHA. Therefore, we are largely dependent on DHA, which is highest in fatty fish such as wild-caught salmon, and also in eggs and dairy. DHA is important in reducing beta-amyloid plaques, which are abnormal protein deposits in the brain and a hallmark of Alzheimer's. Eicosapentaenoic acid (EPA) is another omega-3, found in fatty fish, that is important for cellular activity and a healthy cardiovascular system.

We are able to manufacture some antioxidants, but we also get many of these from foods, especially fruits and vegetables.

Vitamins that protect our brain include the following:

- vitamin A
- vitamin B_1 (thiamine)
- vitamin B_5 (pantothenic acid)
- vitamin B_6
- vitamin B_9 (folate)
- vitamin B_{12}
- vitamin C
- vitamin D
- vitamin E
- vitamin K
- choline (a nutrient with vitamin-like properties)

These vitamins serve many purposes—as antioxidants and anti-inflammatories, and as nutrients that ensure the brain gets what it needs. These important brain vitamins are linked to improved cognitive function, memory, mental clarity, and response time.

Minerals that protect the brain include these:

- iron
- magnesium
- manganese
- potassium
- selenium
- zinc

The minerals provide antioxidant protection in addition to their regulatory function in nerve processes and plaque buildup in the brain. These important trace elements are linked to improved attention and concentration, cognitive function, and response time.

On the Western Diet

The term "Western diet" is used to describe our modern way of eating in the United States. The diet is high in fat, cholesterol, protein, sugar, and salt. Also referred to as the "meat-sweet diet," it includes foods such as high-fat and processed meats, sugary drinks, sweets, and fast foods, many of which are loaded with high-fructose corn syrup or other added sugar, sodium, and trans fats, and contain few antioxidants, vitamins, and minerals. This way of eating promotes obesity, metabolic syndrome, cardiovascular diseases, and (probably) types of dementias, including Alzheimer's disease.

In addition to the links discussed throughout this chapter between inflammation and disease, several studies also link high levels of sodium intake and low levels of physical activity with a reduction in cognitive abilities. What's more, researchers at Oregon Health & Science University find that people who consume diets high in trans fats score lower on thinking and memory tests and experience brain shrinkage similar to that seen in Alzheimer's disease.

As dietitians, we generally don't talk about "bad" foods. All foods can fit into a healthy diet, especially if you subscribe to the 80:20 rule—80 percent of your foods come from nutrient-dense plant-based foods, and 20 percent consist of small portions of foods that are not plant-based.

Inflammation and the Brain

When the body's immune system attacks things it doesn't recognize, such as bacteria, plant pollen, or specific chemicals, it responds with inflammation. This is your body's way of protecting itself. When inflammation persists day in and day out, however, it becomes the enemy.

Inflammation in the brain plays a major role in the progression of Alzheimer's disease. One of the markers for inflammation in the body is a non-protein amino acid called homocysteine. The risk of developing Alzheimer's is strongly linked to your level of homocysteine. The lower your level of it throughout life, the lower your risk of developing serious memory decline. High levels of homocysteine can damage the medial temporal lobe—the area of the brain that rapidly degenerates in Alzheimer's disease. Homocysteine testing is simple and can be done at the doctor's office.

One of the most powerful tools to combat inflammation comes from the grocery store. Homocysteine levels tend to be higher in people whose diets are high in animal protein. Diets that resemble the Mediterranean diet—those high in vegetables, fruits, nuts, fatty fish, olive oil, whole grains, and beans—help the body reduce homocysteine levels. Consuming foods high in folic acid and other B vitamins may also lower homocysteine levels.

There are particular vegetables and fruits (discussed further in later chapters) that are naturally high in antioxidants and compounds called polyphenols, which provide brain protection. The range of colors we see in produce is from polyphenols. Beyond imparting the red to strawberries and the orange to carrots, polyphenols perform the most important work of protecting plants from disease and other environmental threats. They are a type of *phytochemical* (active chemical compound) found in plant foods such as spices, fruits, vegetables, seeds, and legumes. Recently, polyphenols have been getting more attention as scientists have uncovered their antioxidant properties and their potential protective and curative effect on inflammation, chronic disease, and life-threatening human illnesses. They may provide significant protection against neurodegenerative diseases such as Alzheimer's and dementia. Here is a visual guide to fruits and vegetables by color and phytochemical.

Color	Brain-Friendly Produce	Phytochemicals
Red	Beets, cherries, pomegranate, raspberries, red bell pepper, strawberries, tomatoes	Anthocyanins, flavonoids, fiber, carotenoids
Orange and Yellow	Apricots, carrots, citrus, pumpkins, sweet potatoes, turmeric, winter squash	Anthocyanins, carotenoids, fiber, flavonoids, curcumin
Green	Arugula, beet greens, chard, collard greens, dandelion greens, kale, mint, napa cabbage, spinach, thyme	Anthocyanins, apigenin, carotenoids, chlorophyll, flavonoids, isoflavones, insoles, luteolin
Blue and Purple	blueberries, blackberries, cherries, eggplant, plums, grapes	Anthocyanins, catechins, flavonoids, kaempferols, lignans, fiber, quercetins, resveratrol

The Gut–Brain Axis

You might be surprised to learn that your gut is not the same thing as your stomach. In fact, the gut, or the gastrointestinal (GI) tract, stretches all the way from the mouth to the anus. The gut and the brain are connected physically and chemically, and the connection is a two-way street. For example, when stress affects your brain and your emotions, it can cause diarrhea or stomach upset. Likewise, when your stomach or bowels are upset, that may result in emotional distress.

The gut–brain relationship occurs through the central nervous system and gut microbes (tens of trillions of microorganisms and bacteria, many of which are beneficial) in your intestines. Many of these bacteria produce brain-altering substances that can influence the brain and central nervous system by controlling inflammation and hormone production.

An altered microbe population in the gut has been observed in people with Alzheimer's. Two of the key features of Alzheimer's are the development of:

- amyloidosis, which is the accumulation of amyloid-ß (Aß) peptides in the brain
- inflammation of the microglia, brain cells that perform immune system functions in the central nervous system

The buildup of these peptides into plaques plays a central role in the onset of Alzheimer's, while the severity of inflammation in the brain is believed to influence the rate of cognitive decline. In a healthy diet, certain probiotics (helpful bacteria) may reduce amyloidosis and inflammation; research continues in this area.

This chapter provides basic information about Alzheimer's disease, nutrition, and the disease–diet connection. The knowledge you gain here can be powerful as you start to understand your personal risks and begin the development of a prevention plan. The next chapter will review popular brain-healthy diets and provide recommendations for types and amounts of foods to include in your personalized brain-enhancing eating plan.

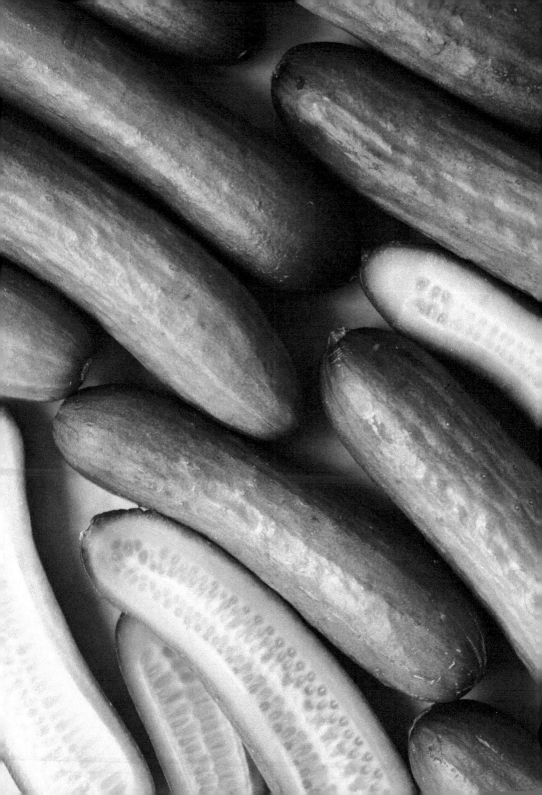

Chapter 2
Brain-Boosting Diets in Perspective

P oor nutritional habits have been linked to reduced brain function. For this reason, several diets have been promoted for their positive effects on the brain and for decreasing the risk factors that can lead to the development of Alzheimer's disease. This chapter will look at some of the most popular diets, the evidence-based research behind them, and our dietary recommendations based upon this research.

Evidence-Based Diets for Brain Health

There are three diets in particular that have received significant press for their Alzheimer's prevention benefits. We briefly review them here, as well as discuss their commonalities and differences.

The Mediterranean Diet

The Mediterranean diet is a modern diet introduced in the 1940s to prevent heart disease. It is based on the dietary patterns of Italy, Greece, and Spain.

The Mediterranean diet may improve cholesterol and blood sugar levels and overall blood vessel health—all factors that have been linked to slowing the rate of cognitive decline, reducing the risk of mild cognitive impairment, and reducing the overall risk of dementia. Recent studies suggest that the Mediterranean diet may function to protect the brain from shrinking. Another study goes so far as to predict that following a Mediterranean diet closely could reduce the likelihood of developing Alzheimer's disease by 54 percent.

The Mediterranean diet guidelines recommend that we eat the following:

- healthy fats like olive oil and the elimination of unhealthy fat sources like butter and margarine
- herbs and spices more often in place of salt, to reduce sodium intake
- primarily plant-based foods such as vegetables, fruits, whole grains, legumes, and nuts
- fish and poultry a few times per week
- moderate amounts of dairy products (mostly as cheese and yogurt)
- red meat no more than a couple of times per month

Dining with others is also encouraged, which fits well with the (optional) recommendation to enjoy a glass of red wine each day.

The MIND Diet

MIND is an acronym for Mediterranean-DASH Intervention for Neurodegenerative Delay. The MIND diet was developed by researchers at the Rush University Medical Center in 2015 following research published in 2014 and 2015. The diet is a combination of the DASH (Dietary Approaches to Stop Hypertension) and Mediterranean diets. The Mediterranean diet was discussed on the previous page. The DASH diet is a lifelong eating approach to prevent and treat high blood pressure (hypertension). DASH is a low-sodium diet that focuses on vegetables, fruits, and low-fat dairy foods and includes moderate amounts of whole grains, fish, poultry, and nuts. The MIND diet singles out foods from both the Mediterranean and DASH diets that are specifically beneficial for brain health.

The MIND diet has been used in a few studies to specifically show its effects on Alzheimer's and brain function. One Rush University study concluded that the MIND diet, when followed closely, lowered the risk of Alzheimer's disease by 53 percent compared to the DASH diet, which lowered risk by 39 percent. Even when the MIND diet was not strictly followed, it lowered the risk of Alzheimer's by 35 percent.

The 10 healthy brain foods outlined in the MIND diet contain many antioxidants and healthy fatty acids: green leafy vegetables, all other vegetables, nuts, berries, beans, whole grains, fish, poultry, olive oil, and wine.

Additionally, there are five unhealthy-brain food groups: red meat, butter or margarine, cheese, pastries and sweets, and fried or fast foods. Consuming these foods is discouraged.

The MIND Diet guidelines recommend that we eat the following:

- at least three servings of whole grains per day
- one salad and at least one other vegetable per day
- at least one serving of beans and one of nuts per day
- at least two servings of poultry per week
- one serving of fish per week
- at least two servings of berries a week

The MIND diet also encourages drinking a glass of red or white wine per day.

The Ketogenic Diet

The ketogenic diet was developed in the 1920s and has been used primarily to treat epilepsy and certain metabolic conditions identified at birth. More recently, it has regained attention as a diet to promote weight loss and continues to be studied for its link to exercise performance, insulin sensitivity, and other health conditions. The diet is very restricted in carbohydrates and therefore can be challenging to follow long term.

The ketogenic diet shows some promise related to insulin sensitivity, glucose tolerance, inflammation reduction, and a reduction of damaging protein plaques. However, evidence-based research is limited and currently inconclusive regarding the ketogenic diet's effect on Alzheimer's risk. Ketosis, a process where the body burns fat instead of carbohydrates for energy, does not occur if the diet is not strictly followed.

This diet plan promotes 70 to 90 percent fat consumption and extremely limited carbohydrate intake—only 20 to 50 grams per day (1 large banana contains about 30 grams of carbohydrates, for example). Since the consumption of carbohydrates is limited, the diet is centered on eating the following:

- foods that are very high in fat, such as meat, cheese, butter and cream, fatty fish, eggs, nuts, and seeds
- very low-carbohydrate vegetables

Fruit, grains, and legumes are excluded from the diet. Since the macronutrient distribution of this diet is significantly restricted, risks of nutritional deficiency exist and supplements are required. Special attention should be paid to fiber, calcium, iron, folic acid, and vitamin D.

For these reasons and until further evidence-based research exists, we do not recommend following the ketogenic diet to promote brain health.

The Common Links

The Mediterranean and MIND diets are both plant-based, and both recommend significant consumption of vegetables, fruits, legumes, beans, and whole grains. Similar to the Mediterranean diet, the MIND diet encourages poultry at least twice per week and fish once per week. Both diets allow for an abundance of low-carbohydrate vegetables as well as nuts and seeds. All three diets allow wine consumption, with the ketogenic diet restricting use within daily total carbohydrate parameters. All of these diets restrict high-sugar foods, which can cause higher insulin levels and lead to inflammation in brain tissue, resulting in the brain secreting the damaging beta amyloid linked to Alzheimer's disease. Each diet can also be relatively low calorie, depending upon serving sizes.

Alternative Brain Fuel

Glucose (from carbohydrates) is the body's favorite form of fuel to burn for energy. If carbohydrates are taken out of the diet or severely restricted, the brain must use an alternative fuel source in order to function properly. This process, called ketogenesis, converts fat to that new fuel source—ketones—to be used for energy.

The extremely low-carbohydrate ketogenic diet has been successfully used to treat epilepsy for years. Research is underway to assess the benefit of the ketogenic diet (and variations of the traditional diet) in other diseases such as Alzheimer's, but the only testing done by the end of 2016 has been uncontrolled studies, observation studies, and anecdotal evidence.

Although the mechanisms for future research studies are not yet defined, researchers will be looking at a few leads for how using ketones as a fuel source may help combat Alzheimer's:

- Brown University neuropathologists identified the brain's inability to effectively utilize glucose in the brains of people with cognitive loss (implying improvements in brain function with ketones as the fuel source), and they have pegged Alzheimer's as type 3 diabetes.
- Animal models show ketone bodies have an antioxidant effect and reduce inflammation. Even when a very low-carbohydrate diet was combined with saturated fats, there was a decrease in harmful protein deposits in the brain.
- Some reported improvements in memory and brain function have been reported in both animals and humans following implementation of a ketogenic diet.

Dietary Differences

The following chart shows the main differences in the diets.

	Mediterranean Diet	MIND Diet	Ketogenic Diet
Primary goal	Prevention of chronic disease (cardiovascular and other) and increased longevity	Prevention of cognitive decline	Treatment of epilepsy and certain metabolic conditions; now popular for weight loss
Vegetables	3 to 4 servings or more daily	Vegetables encouraged and at least one leafy green salad daily	Very low-carb vegetables allowed within daily carb intake levels
Fruit	Encouraged—consumed as dessert or snacks	Berries encouraged	Not allowed, except berries allowed within daily carb intake levels
Whole grains, legumes, and nuts	Encouraged	Encouraged	No whole grains or legumes allowed; nuts encouraged
Meats	Red meat rarely; poultry and eggs allowed in moderation	Poultry allowed	All meats allowed, including high-fat and processed
Fish	2 or more servings per week	At least one serving per week	Fatty fishes encouraged
Olive oil	Daily use recommended; use as primary fat	Daily use recommended; use as primary fat	Recommended
Butter and margarine	Small amounts of butter allowed; margarine discouraged	Discouraged; less than 1 tablespoon daily	All fats allowed and encouraged
Dairy products	Cheese and yogurt allowed in moderation	Cheese and yogurt allowed in moderation	Allowed within daily carb intake levels
Red wine	Moderate consumption: no more than 1 glass daily for women and 2 for men	1 glass a day allowed	Allowed within daily carb intake levels

According to the Rush University study, people with a higher intake of MIND foods showed slower cognitive decline compared to those on the Mediterranean diet, even though the Mediterranean diet slowed the decline as well. Evidence-based research shows that diets promoting antioxidants, phytochemicals, and omega-3 fatty acids increase brain health. The ketogenic diet's impact on Alzheimer's disease is still being researched.

Putting It All Together

The following food categories and serving recommendations have been established to help guide you in the types and amounts of brain-healthy foods to eat each day. It is important to note that foods excluded from this guidebook may not be unhealthy or harmful but rather are either too numerous to include (as in the case of hundreds of different vegetables and fruits from around the world) or not supported by scientific research.

A good "rule of brain" is to fill at least three-quarters of your plate with brain-nourishing leafy greens and other colorful vegetables, fruits, legumes, and whole grains. The remaining quarter of your plate can include fish or protein alternatives, nuts, seeds, healthy extras, and occasionally a favorite food not considered brain nourishing. Fresh, local, organic, and in-season foods often provide the highest nutrient content and lowest risk of contaminants; however, it is better to eat the foods from this guide in any form rather than not at all.

Spices/Herbs

While spices and herbs have been used for health purposes for centuries, today's consumers are generally unfamiliar with many of them, and spice shelves across America—both in homes and in grocery stores—are cluttered with bottles of who-knows-how-old spices. All spices and herbs originate from roots, fruits, flowers, seeds, barks, or leaves and are high in an array of vitamins, minerals, and antioxidants. Those reviewed in this guidebook are just an introduction to the numerous spices and herbs that are worth revisiting as we search for clues to the prevention of Alzheimer's disease. Consider growing your own herb garden or drying your own spices to have the freshest access year-round.

> **Recommended servings**
> Ditch the salt shaker and consider using at least one brain-healthy spice or herb at every meal.
> **What is a serving size?**
> Recommended amounts are not available. Chop, zest, sprinkle, and use according to your taste. As a general rule, use three times the amount of fresh versus dried herbs.

Leafy Greens

What's not to love about leafy greens? These vegetables are perhaps the least controversial food in existence, with an overabundance of healthy components to improve brain health. While all leafy greens are healthy, in this guidebook we have included a few of the most nutritious. Low in calories, they are chock-full of flavor in addition to fiber; folic acid; vitamins A, C, and K; magnesium; potassium; and a host of phytochemicals, all of which have been studied regarding their positive role in maintaining a healthy mind. In several large studies, the consumption of leafy greens resulted in the largest reduction of cardiovascular risk, which is believed to equate to a lowered risk of developing Alzheimer's.

Recommended servings
One or more servings daily
What is a serving size?
2 cups raw or 1 cup cooked

Other Vegetables

If they are prepared in a healthy way (including leaving the skins on), it's nearly impossible to eat too many vegetables. Veggies are naturally low in sodium, calories, and fat; contain zero cholesterol; and are packed with brain-enhancing nutrients such as folic acid; vitamins A, C, and K; potassium; and fiber. Cruciferous vegetables, such as cauliflower, cabbage, broccoli, and Brussels sprouts, have been associated with a reduced rate of cognitive decline. In addition to Alzheimer's prevention, increased consumption of vegetables results in the reduced risk of hypertension, heart disease, type 2 diabetes, some types of cancer, and obesity.

Recommended servings
Four or more servings daily; two or three different colors (eat the rainbow); keep the skin/peel on if possible
What is a serving size?
1 cup

Fruit

Skins and all, fruit is serious business when it comes to Alzheimer's prevention. In a study published in the *American Journal of Medicine*, of the 2,000 Japanese-American participants, those who drank at least three glasses of fruit or vegetable juice per week had a 76 percent decrease in their probable risk of Alzheimer's versus those who drank less than one glass per week. The positive effects are thought to be related to the high amounts of polyphenols in the fruits and vegetables, mostly found in the skin and peels. The risk of developing Alzheimer's disease is greatly reduced in those individuals who eat two or more servings of fruit daily; this risk reduction may also be associated with fruits' high content of folate and vitamin B_6, which lower homocysteine levels.

> **Recommended servings**
> Three servings daily; two or three different colors
> (eat the rainbow); keep the skin/peel on if possible
> **What is a serving size?**
> One small piece of fruit or ½ cup

Legumes

Also known as pulses, legumes are an economical plant food packed with protein, fiber, magnesium, and B vitamins, all of which are essential for a healthy brain. They have no saturated fat, and they help you feel full, which may contribute to obesity prevention. Within this group are beans, peas, garbanzos, lupines (such as peanuts), and lentils; thousands of different species of legumes are grown around the world. If you are using canned legumes, drain and rinse them before eating to reduce sodium intake. Choosing to cook from dry legumes preserves the most nutrients. The legumes reviewed in this guidebook contribute to brain nourishment and reduce inflammation due to their super high amounts of phyto-chemicals with antioxidant properties.

Recommended servings
One serving daily is ideal, with a minimum of three to four servings per week
What is a serving size?
½ cup cooked

Whole Grains

We would like to introduce you to a variety of whole grains in this category, some of which are eaten more routinely in countries with lower incidence of Alzheimer's disease. Unlike refined grains, which have been stripped of their bran and germ, whole grains are just as they sound: whole. With all of their parts intact, whole grains are a great source of the powerful antioxidant vitamin E, as well as many B vitamins, magnesium, selenium, and a significant amount of fiber. Impressive research has identified a much lower early death rate among individuals who eat a significant amount (two to six servings a day) of whole grains.

Recommended servings
At least three servings daily
What is a serving size?
½ cup cooked grains or 1 ounce whole grain equivalent (see choosemyplate.gov/grains for suggestions)

Nuts and Seeds

Eating a handful of nuts and/or seeds a day might just be the ticket to keeping your brain healthy. Tree nuts and seeds from a variety of sources are counted in this category. (Peanuts are actually a legume, so you will find them in that grouping of foods.) The fiber, protein, and fat in nuts and seeds provide a feeling of fullness, which may help prevent overeating and obesity. The components of nuts and seeds also lower total cholesterol and LDLs (the harmful form of cholesterol), which in turn reduces the risk of Alzheimer's disease. Some varieties of nuts and seeds are higher in omega-3 fatty acids than others, while some are higher in antioxidant-rich vitamin E, and still others are higher in selenium, an important nutrient in brain communication.

> **Recommended servings**
> At least one serving daily
> **What is a serving size?**
> ¼ cup nuts, 1½ tablespoons nut butter, 2 tablespoons seeds, or 1 ounce equivalent (see choosemyplate.gov/protein-foods)

Oils

The two oils recommended in this category—extra-virgin olive oil and coconut oil—are very different in their chemical makeup and also the ways in which they may be helpful to the brain and Alzheimer's prevention. While extra-virgin olive oil (a monoun-saturated fatty acid) has been studied extensively in relationship to inflammation, cell regeneration, and potential reduction in Alzheimer's disease, the role of coconut oil is still in its research infancy. In theory, it is thought that coconut oil, a saturated fat, may provide an alternative energy source to the brain. This would result in the reduction of damage caused by using glucose as a fuel source, as well as improved brain function. Clinical trials to test this theory are currently underway in the United States.

Recommended servings
Extra-virgin olive oil: at least one serving daily
Coconut oil: recommended amounts are not available
What is a serving size?
2 tablespoons or ⅛ cup

Proteins

The protein foods recommended in this guidebook—eggs, fatty fish, and tofu—stand out for their contribution to a healthy brain. They provide a bevy of nutrients with positive effects on the mind. A number of those nutrients—omega-3 fatty acids, selenium, vitamin D, and choline—are especially beneficial in lowering Alzheimer's disease risk, maintaining neurotransmitters in the brain, and improving cognitive function and memory skills.

Some fish contain more mercury than others and should be eaten with caution, especially if you are pregnant, trying to become pregnant, or breastfeeding. Large fish such as king mackerel and bigeye tuna have consistently reported higher mercury contamination, while many other varieties of mackerel and tuna have lower amounts.

Recommended servings
At least one food from this category daily
Three or four servings of fish per week
What is a serving size?
3 to 4 ounces fish
6 ounces tofu

Fermented Foods

It is no surprise that the ancient practice of fermenting foods and beverages has potential brain-boosting effects. The connection between the human microbiome and the mind is becoming increasingly clear: the antioxidant and anti-inflammatory effects of fermented foods aid in brain neurotransmission, glycemic control, and many other pathways that hold a key to Alzheimer's disease prevention. The fermented foods featured on our list are full of probiotics and a plethora of mind-enhancing nutrients.

Recommended servings

One serving daily

What is a serving size?

½ to 1 cup fermented foods; 1 tablespoon apple cider vinegar

Others

In the "others" category are three items that deserve recognition in the area of brain health: coffee, green tea, and seaweed. While not everyone reacts in the same way to each, there is a fair amount of research showing the positive effects of coffee and caffeine on the brains of Alzheimer's patients. Green tea and seaweed contain abundant amounts of antioxidants, the damage-erasing components of cognitive function.

Recommended servings

Coffee and/or green tea: at least one serving daily

Seaweed: one serving per week

What is a serving size?

1 cup coffee or green tea

½ cup seaweed

A WORD ON

Meat and Dairy

Meat—chicken, turkey, beef, pork, and lamb—as well as many dairy foods not listed in this guidebook can fit into your meal plan. Independently, these foods do not have the nutritional profile to make the cut as brain-healthy foods, mostly due to their high amounts of saturated fat. However, they contribute essential nutrients to the diet and can fit nicely into a food plan that will nourish your brain.

In addition to being a great source of protein, meat and dairy foods provide a significant source of homocysteine-lowering vitamin B_{12}. Studies show that when B vitamin–rich foods are combined with omega-3 fatty acids, improved memory function and less brain shrinkage results. This helps support the consumption of fatty fish, nuts, and seeds as a main protein source for those wishing to promote brain health. Controlling portion sizes, using meat and dairy foods as a flavoring versus making them the center of the plate, and combining them with vegetables, legumes, and herbs may just be the winning combination for those who wish to nourish their brains for the long-term. See chapter 4 for ways to incorporate animal proteins in your meal plan.

Evidence-Based Brain Food

While this chart is by no means comprehensive, it should help you get a good start on stocking your kitchen and filling your plate with foods that the evidence has shown to be healthy for the brain.

Spices	Cacao, cardamom, ginger, mint, turmeric
Leafy Greens	Arugula, collard greens, kale, spinach, watercress
Other Vegetables	Beets, broccoli, Brussels sprouts, garlic, red cabbage, winter squash
Fruit	Berries, cherries, citrus, grapes, pomegranates
Legumes	Beans, black-eyed peas, lentils, peanuts, soybeans
Whole Grains	Barley, brown rice, buckwheat, farro, oats
Nuts/Seeds	Almonds, chia seeds, flaxseeds, pistachios, walnuts
Oils	Extra-virgin olive oil, coconut oil
Proteins	Eggs, salmon, tofu, trout, whitefish
Fermented Foods	Kefir, miso, red wine, sauerkraut, yogurt
Others	Coffee, green tea, seaweed

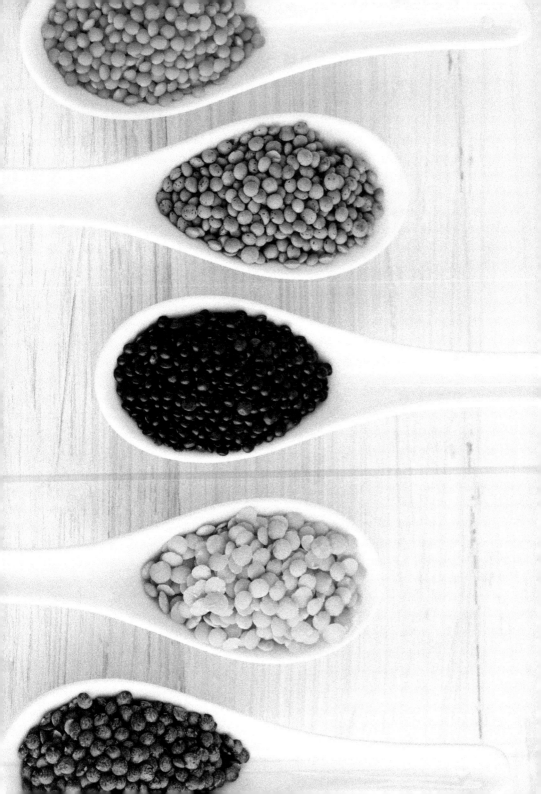

Chapter 3
Foods that Nourish and Protect the Brain

Our message for Alzheimer's prevention is simple: Eat more brain foods. The more than 100 recommended foods in this guide have been compiled from multiple studies published in the United States and other countries, all of which are listed in the book's bibliography. While there is no one diet or food proven to prevent Alzheimer's disease, there is evidence, as noted in chapters 1 and 2, that diet may decrease the risk of developing Alzheimer's. What we *can* say with certainty is that the foods in this guide contain properties that are beneficial to healthy brain function. When combined into a generally healthy diet, they have great promise for preserving brain health over the years. Chapter 4 will show you how to move from knowing about these foods to incorporating them into a healthy diet.

For a quick scan of the more than 100 brain foods profiled in this chapter, see the table on page 46. This chapter offers profiles of each of these foods, organized by the categories we outlined in chapter 2. Each brain food listed has mind-health attributes and studies supporting its connection to Alzheimer's prevention. A brief description of the nutrients, associated research, and ways in which the food promotes the health of the brain is included.

Each brain food profile also notes one or more contributions the food makes toward brain health; these contributions are categorized into the following 11 areas:

- Anti-inflammatory
- Brain response time
- Cognitive function
- Concentration (focus)
- Cell regeneration
- Memory
- Mental clarity
- Nerve function
- Nerve growth
- Reasoning
- Sleep enhancement

In addition, you will find more in-depth features on 10 of the foods. These 10 deserve special recognition for their role as brain-health powerhouses. While some foods profiled in this chapter will be familiar, a few may not. We hope you will give each and every one of them a try!

SPICES AND HERBS

Basil

This highly fragrant herb has been used in Mediterranean cuisine for centuries. Basil has strong antioxidant properties and an enzyme-inhibiting effect that qualifies it as a great anti-inflammatory food. One teaspoon of dried basil is thought to have the equivalent antioxidant potency to a cup of nourishing sweet potatoes. To get the most from its strong flavors, plentiful anti-oxidants, and vitamins A, C, and K, try using fresh basil in salads and vinaigrettes.

- Anti-inflammatory
- Cognitive function

Black Pepper

Black pepper may be the second most utilized spice in US kitchens, right behind its less nourishing partner, salt. The active ingredient in black pepper, piperine, has been shown to improve cognitive function (attention and focus) in the brain. Black pepper also lends a helping hand to the brain-powerhouse spice turmeric. When consumed together, piperine has been found to enhance the absorption of curcumin (turmeric's brain booster) by 2,000 percent.

- Anti-inflammatory
- Cognitive function
- Concentration

Cacao

Chocolate is made from cacao beans. The darker the chocolate (more cacao), the higher the antioxidant content; the higher the antioxidants, the lower the risk of brain and dementia issues. Various studies have shown that consuming a cacao beverage daily for a month was associated with significant improvements in cognitive function and blood flow in the brain. This is due to the high level of flavonols in dark chocolate. For more information on this powerful brain food, see the next page.

- Anti-inflammatory
- Cognitive function
- Nerve function

Cardamom

This spice is a relative of ginger and turmeric and has antioxidant properties that help protect brain cells from free radical damage. It also contains B vitamins, which may boost energy and recall. For a new twist to old favorites, add it to baked goods, tea or coffee, stews, and curries.

- Anti-inflammatory
- Memory
- Nerve function

Chamomile

Chamomile is the common name for several daisy-like plants often used in herbal infusions such as tea. Chamomile contains luteolin, a flavonoid that has been found to improve brain function in the hippocampus area of the brain—the center for memory and learning. Chamomile blends well with licorice or mint for a double brain boost.

- Anti-inflammatory
- Cognitive function
- Memory
- Sleep enhancement

Cilantro

Also known as coriander or Chinese parsley, cilantro is a flavorful herb that adds zest to many Mexican and Thai dishes. It pairs especially well with eggs, fish, and beans. Cilantro is thought to have antioxidant and lipid-lowering effects. It is high in vitamins A and K and contains an enzyme to help break down complex

Cacao

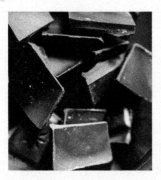

Does dark chocolate provide a sweet treat for your brain? Indeed! All chocolate comes from cacao (or cocoa) beans. In its raw form, cacao is the purest form of chocolate you can consume. Not just any chocolate will do for your brain, though. Milk chocolate contains less cacao by weight than does dark chocolate. The process by which dark chocolate is changed to milk chocolate can lower the amount of brain-nourishing flavonols by 60 to 90 percent.

- Limited clinical trials show an improvement in attention, cognitive function, and memory with the consumption of cacao flavonols (antioxidant compounds found in cacao). One Harvard study found that people who drank two cups of a hot chocolate drink a day had improved memory and blood flow to the brain.
- Cacao is much less processed than cocoa powder or chocolate bars, and because of this, it is chock-full of anti-oxidants. Cacao also contains the brain-healthy nutrients potassium and magnesium.

Consuming a dark chocolate cocoa drink or a snack with cacao in it may not only be beneficial to reduce your risk of Alzheimer's disease but may also satisfy your sweet tooth. Try adding it to pudding and granola bars or sprinkle it over fruit.

When selecting chocolate, choose 85 percent cocoa or more—the darker the chocolate, the better it is for your brain.

carbohydrates—all of which are significant for brain health. Cilantro is one of several herbs able to retain their strong anti-oxidant capacity even when dried.

• Anti-inflammatory   • Nerve function

Cinnamon

This ancient spice may hold some secrets to Alzheimer's prevention. Besides delivering anti-inflammatory benefits, cinnamon also contains compounds thought to improve communication between brain cells as well as interfere with the buildup of damaging tau proteins in the brain. Cinnamon is linked to lowered blood sugars and reduced heart disease risk factors, and provides a plethora of other impressive health benefits.

• Anti-inflammatory   • Memory   • Concentration

Cumin

After black pepper, cumin is the most commonly used spice in the world (excluding the United States) and is widely used in countries with low Alzheimer's rates. It is a wonderful addition to curry powder and is delicious in Mexican or Middle Eastern dishes. Cumin is a good source of magnesium, and it shows promise in boosting learning capacity in the brain and preventing cognitive decline.

• Cognitive function   • Memory   • Concentration

Ginger

Popular in Asian and Indian cuisines, this sweet-spicy root is a common home remedy for nausea but also shows amazing promise in dementia prevention. It is both a potent anti-inflammatory and antioxidant, making it a very effective food for preventing Alzheimer's disease. Ginger has been shown to provide some protection against the buildup of beta-amyloid proteins in the brain. It can easily be incorporated into the diet through seasonings, salad dressings, or even brewed into tea.

• Anti-inflammatory   • Memory

Horseradish

This potent root has multiple qualities that make it a great brain food. Horseradish contains dietary fiber, vitamin C, folate and other B vitamins, and antioxidants. Certain active compounds found in horseradish have anti-inflammatory and nerve-soothing effects. The hot, sharp flavor of this root pairs well with fish, seafood, leafy greens, and tomatoes.

• Anti-inflammatory   • Nerve function

Lavender

Lavender creates a calming and soporific effect, which can improve sleep patterns, an important factor in the prevention of Alzheimer's disease. Its anti-inflammatory effect has a positive impact on blood pressure reduction. While lavender has been studied mostly as an essential oil, it has started to gain popularity in the United States as a cooking ingredient—used as an infusion in drinks and desserts or mixed with other brain-powerhouse spices like rosemary and thyme in herbes de Provence.

• Anti-inflammatory   • Sleep enhancement

Brain Foods by Category

Spices and Herbs

Basil	Cilantro	Lavender	Rosemary
Black Pepper	Cinnamon	Licorice	Sage
Cacao	Cumin	Mint	Thyme
Cardamom	Ginger	Nutmeg	Turmeric
Chamomile	Horseradish	Parsley	Wasabi

Leafy Greens

Arugula	Collard Greens	Kale	Spinach
Beet Greens	Dandelion Greens	Napa Cabbage	Watercress
Chard			

Other Vegetables

Artichokes	Cauliflower	Leeks	Shiitake
Asparagus	Chile Peppers	Okra	Mushrooms
Avocados	Cucumbers	Onions	Sweet Potatoes
Beets	Eggplant	Potatoes	Tomatoes
Broccoli	Garlic	Pumpkins	Winter Squash
Brussels Sprouts	Jicama	Red Bell Peppers	Yams
Carrots	Kohlrabi	Red Cabbage	Zucchini

Fruit

Apricots	−Cranberries	Cherries	Melons
Berries:	−Marionberries	Citrus	Plantains
−Blackberries	−Raspberries	Grapes	Plums
−Blueberries	−Strawberries	Mangos	Pomegranates

Legumes

Beans	Garbanzo Beans	Lentils	Peanuts
Black-Eyed Peas	(Chickpeas)	Mung Beans	Soybeans

Whole Grains

Amaranth	Buckwheat	Millet	Spelt
Barley	Bulgur	Oats	Wheat Germ
Brown Rice	Farro		

Nuts/Seeds

Almonds	Flaxseeds	Pecans	Pumpkin Seeds
Chia Seeds	Hazelnuts	Pistachios	Walnuts

Oils

Coconut Oil	Extra-Virgin Olive Oil

Proteins

Eggs	–Butterfish	–Herring	–Tuna
Fish:	–Carp	–Lake Trout	–Whitefish
–American	–Chilean	–Mackerel	–Wild Salmon
Shad	Sea Bass	–Sablefish	Tofu
–Anchovies	–Eel	–Sardines	

Fermented Foods

Apple Cider Vinegar	Craft Beer	Miso	Sauerkraut
	Kefir	Red Wine	Yogurt

Other

Coffee	Green Tea	Seaweed

Licorice

Licorice root is widely used as a flavoring in sweets and beverages such as craft beer and tea. It contains brain-bolstering B vitamins, choline, magnesium, and selenium as well as a host of polyphenols (bioactive plant compounds that make possible antioxidant action in the brain). Due to its potency and some medication interactions, please check with your doctor before using natural licorice.

• Anti-inflammatory   • Cognitive function

Mint

This refreshing plant is easily incorporated into a diet by serving it in beverages, on lamb, in soups, or mixed into fresh fruit or vegetable salads. It is one of the most powerful antioxidants found among plants, containing many vitamins and minerals such as vitamins A and C, magnesium, and potassium. Mint is anti-inflammatory, as well. This combination of nutrients is a surefire hit for Alzheimer's prevention.

• Anti-inflammatory   • Memory

Nutmeg

Grown on a species of evergreen tree, nutmeg is an aromatic spice often found in holiday cooking, baked into sweets, added to the top of a dish as a garnish, or blended into a marinade or dry rub. It is a powerful antioxidant and has been used in traditional Chinese medicine to relieve pain. It is rich in B-complex vitamins such as folic acid and riboflavin, and contains vitamin C as well, all of which contribute to an Alzheimer's prevention plan.

• Anti-inflammatory   • Cognitive function   • Memory

Parsley

Although often used as a garnish, parsley could potentially fit into the leafy green category given all its potent mind-nourishing antioxidants. One such antioxidant, luteolin (a flavonoid), has been found to improve brain function in the hippocampus, the area in the brain known to be the center for memory and learning.

- Anti-inflammatory
- Concentration
- Memory

Rosemary

One of the most popular herbs in the world, rosemary is used in cooking and herbal teas. Consumption of rosemary has been linked to improved focus, speed, and accuracy on cognitive testing. It is heavily used as part of the Mediterranean diet, is a natural antioxidant, and has been used to extend the shelf life of perishable foods.

- Anti-inflammatory
- Concentration
- Reasoning
- Brain response time
- Nerve function

Sage

There is promising evidence suggesting that sage, derived from the Latin word *salvare* or "to save," may improve mood and mental performance in healthy young people, and boost memory and attention in older adults. Sage, a member of the mint family, inhibits the release of enzymes that break down communicators in the brain. One study showed sage extract fared well in enhancing learning and cognition in older adults with mild to moderate Alzheimer's disease.

- Anti-inflammatory
- Concentration
- Cognitive function
- Memory

Foods Worth Searching For

Although they are not well known or commonly found on the shelves of the supermarket, the following foods show great promise for their contribution to brain health. These foods are either currently being studied or appear to have what it takes to make them the new up-and-coming brain enhancers. Give them a try!

Ashwagandha Also known as Indian ginseng, poison gooseberry, or winter cherry, ashwagandha is a root with brain-protecting potential. While its berries can be used as a substitute for rennet in cheesemaking, the root is often ground into an herbal supplement or dried and used in teas and other beverages. Studies show it has a cognition-promoting effect and may be useful to control memory deficit as we age. Consider trying it in tea, milk, or hot cereal. As with any herbal remedy, consult your doctor before taking it, to avoid any interactions with medications.

Black Currants Starting in the early 1800s in Europe, black currant extract has been used to treat cold and flu symptoms. Recent research, however, has shown that these sour berries can also help with cognitive function. They contain many of the nutrients linked to Alzheimer's prevention, such as flavonoids, vitamin B_6, polyphenols, vitamin C, iron, and many strong antioxidants. When shopping, specifically look for "black currants" as Zante currants may be sold as an imposter. Fresh currants may be more difficult to find; dried are more generally available.

Hibiscus The beautiful flower of this bushy annual plant is often used in teas, jams, and sauces. Hibiscus is loaded with antioxidants and has been shown to reduce blood pressure in people who drink hibiscus tea for two to six weeks. One particular flavonoid phyto-chemical in hibiscus has been linked to a reduction of tau proteins in the brain (damaging plaque-building proteins found in the brains of Alzheimer's patients). Try hibiscus tea hot or cold, or if you are really daring, the dried flowers are edible and can be used in your favorite dishes or as a garnish.

Kamut This ancient wheat may have brain-boosting nutrition when compared to modern whole wheat. In studies comparing the two, kamut consumption resulted in improvement in inflammatory testing, reduction in total and LDL (bad) cholesterol, and a mild reduction in fasting blood glucose. These laboratory markers are important, as they relate to inflammation in the body, cardiovascular disease, diabetes, and Alzheimer's disease. This sweet, almost but-tery-tasting wheat can be cooked as a hot cereal, served as a side dish, or used in casseroles or soups.

Nut and Seed Oils Walnut oil. Butternut squash oil. Black cumin seed oil. Apricot kernel oil. If fancy finishing oils are something you are interested in experimenting with, the benefits may be more than just unique flavors. Nut and seed oils are high in vitamin D, vitamin E, and omega-3 fatty acids, all of which have been studied for their posi-tive effects on brain health. Walnut oil even has melatonin, adding a sleep benefit. Look for these tasty oils in natural foods co-ops or specialty food stores. Use them in salad dressings, in light sautéing, or even drizzled over vegetables, ice cream, or fruit.

Thyme

Containing two strong antioxidants, vitamins A and C, thyme is linked with improved learning skills and overall maintenance of brain health. A Brazilian study found that one antioxidant in thyme, a flavonoid called apigenin, strengthened connections between neurons and other specialized cells in the brain, which may be helpful in the prevention of Alzheimer's disease. Thyme, with 60 different varieties, pairs well with brain-healthy fish, bean, and egg dishes.

• Anti-inflammatory • Cognitive function • Nerve function

Turmeric

This beautiful yellow spice adds a burst of flavor and color to foods and has been used to treat inflammation for thousands of years. Curcumin, a naturally occurring plant compound found in turmeric, is one of the principal healthy phytochemicals. Curcumin acts to protect the body from oxidative stress and inflammation, which contributes to cell damage, diseases of aging, and declined memory function. For more information on this powerful spice, see the next page.

• Anti-inflammatory • Cognitive function • Memory

Wasabi

This spicy hot root vegetable is related to cabbage, horseradish, and mustard and is commonly served alongside sushi. It is rich in carotenoids (brain-protecting antioxidants converted in the body to vitamin A). Research shows that aside from its anti-inflammatory properties to reduce Alzheimer's risk, it also contains antibacterial and anticancer properties.

• Anti-inflammatory • Cognitive function • Nerve growth

Turmeric

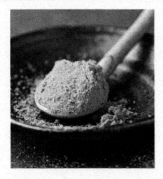

In addition to being a superfood, turmeric has a super pretty color and a super hearty dose of antioxidants! Commonly used in Asian and Middle Eastern foods, this spice has gained popularity in the United States due to its health benefits. Studies show that populations with considerable intakes of turmeric or curry have lower rates of Alzheimer's disease and dementia.

A root from the ginger family, turmeric has been used for centuries as a treatment for inflammatory disorders. Here are some of its benefits:

- Turmeric contains brain healthy phytochemicals, including curcumin, which has been the most-studied phytochemical for its impact on Alzheimer's disease. Curcumin also stimulates the production of DHA from ALA omega-3 fatty acids and inhibits the accumulation of destructive beta-amyloids in the brain.
- One crucial component of turmeric is aromatic-turmerone, which may help in the recovery of brain function.
- Research indicates that eating turmeric and black pepper together may increase the spice's absorption and effectiveness.

Turmeric can be purchased in fresh or dry form. Try adding it to your diet daily in teas, stir-fries, smoothies, eggs, grains, roasted veggies, and soups.

LEAFY GREENS

Arugula

This peppery salad green has more calcium than any other leafy green and is a good source of brain-enhancing nutrients, including vitamin C, beta-carotene, and folate. Its antioxidant powers can help reduce the amounts of damaging materials in the brain that are thought to be linked to Alzheimer's disease. Arugula is a very social green—it is great tossed with spinach or kale and mixed into casseroles, soups, and sautéed vegetables.

• Anti-inflammatory   • Cognitive function   • Nerve function

Beet Greens

These nontraditional greens have made a mark in the nutritional world with their dense nutrient content. They are rich in the phytochemicals flavonoids (antioxidant) and carotenoids (eye health), vitamins A, C, K, and many B-complex members (riboflavin, niacin, folate), as well as potassium. Eating beet greens is an excellent choice to help avoid cognitive decline.

• Anti-inflammatory   • Cognitive function

Chard

Chard is one of the healthiest foods around. It is packed with antioxidant flavonoids and vitamin K—both of which may play a key role in boosting memory and ousting damaging by-products in the brain. Chard is a source of vitamins A and C, and of minerals that protect against cognitive decline and Alzheimer's disease.

• Anti-inflammatory   • Cognitive function   • Memory

Collard Greens

Much like eating its leafy green counterparts, consuming a serving of collard greens a day will help keep dementia away. A 2015 research project funded by the National Institutes of Health studied 954 older individuals over the course of five years. At the end of this time, the team determined that those who routinely consumed one or two servings of leafy greens daily demonstrated the mental capacity of someone more than 10 years younger, compared with those who did not eat leafy greens.

• Anti-inflammatory   • Cognitive function   • Concentration

Dandelion Greens

Not just an annoying weed, these leafy greens are a powerhouse for brain health. They contain a significant amount of vitamin E, which is a free radical fighter that helps prevent brain cell damage. Dandelion greens are full of astounding amounts of vitamins A and K. These nutrients provide a memory boost and are helpful when learning new skills. Caution: Do not harvest dandelion greens if you are unsure whether they have been chemically treated.

• Anti-inflammatory   • Cognitive function   • Memory

Kale

Some people consider kale to be the most potent food on the planet, and they might not be far off. Kale is filled with antioxidants; vitamins A, C, and K; and manganese, all important for brain health. Kale also contains omega-3 fatty acids. The plant-based omega-3 ALA (alpha-linolenic acid) is linked to numerous health benefits, including the lowered risk of Alzheimer's disease. For more information on this powerful brain food, see the next page.

* Anti-Inflammatory   * Cell regeneration   * Nerve function

Napa Cabbage

This delicate and lacy-leafed green vegetable ranks number two on the Centers for Disease Control and Prevention's Powerhouse Fruits and Vegetables list. It's an antioxidant superhero, thanks to polyphenols known as anthocyanins (protective plant compounds), and vitamins C and K. See the spinach, cauliflower, and broccoli profiles for the brain-health attributes also contained in napa cabbage. Each characteristic is important in the prevention or delay of Alzheimer's disease.

* Anti-inflammatory   * Memory
* Concentration   * Nerve growth

Spinach

Green and mighty, spinach is rich in B vitamins such as folate, which regulates homocysteine levels in the blood. Heightened homocysteine levels are seen in patients with Alzheimer's disease. Spinach also contains beta-carotene, a strong antioxidant that prevents the formation of free radicals, and lutein, which decreases the number of oxidized red blood cells in the brain. A study concluded that by consuming one serving of spinach a day, you can help prevent cognitive decline.

* Anti-inflammatory   * Cognitive function   * Memory

Kale

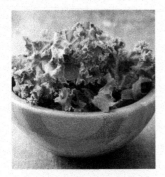

Do you believe the ancient Turkish saying "every leaf of kale you chew adds another stem to your tree of life"? Kale, yeah! It may help you live longer and keep your brain healthy, too.

- Kale is loaded with antioxidants—vitamins A, C, and K. One cup of chopped fresh kale has the vitamin C content of a medium-size orange or grapefruit.
- Kale contains the plant-based omega-3 ALA, which promotes numerous health benefits, including a lowered risk of Alzheimer's disease.
- Due to its vitamin K, beta-carotene, and folate content, kale consumption has been linked to a slowing of cognitive decline in older age.
- Many of kale's top brain-health components are more effective when they are combined with other foods. For example, fats like olive oil and avocado make the carotenoid antioxidants in kale more available for use by the body and brain. One great way to activate these antioxidants is to rub or massage the leaves with olive oil prior to making your salad or kale dish.

Kale can be baked, made into a variety of main or side dishes, and added raw to smoothies or pasta dishes.

Watercress

Topping the Centers for Disease Control and Prevention's Powerhouse Fruits and Vegetables list, this ancient green lost popularity in the nineteenth century, but its benefits have recently been rediscovered. Its abundant quantity of vitamin K helps fight Alzheimer's by increasing calcium regulation in the brain. Its many antioxidants (vitamin A, C, and the three flavonoids) help reduce the damage that inflammation causes in the body. The nitrates found in watercress may lower blood pressure, which reduces the risk for cardiovascular disease and Alzheimer's disease.

• Anti-inflammatory　　　• Cognitive function　　　• Memory

OTHER VEGETABLES

Artichokes

A thistle or a flower? Either way, the artichoke packs a punch with its abundance of vitamin C and other antioxidants, protecting brain cells from damage. Artichokes are a great source of vitamin K, which is linked to brain health by its ability to reduce damage to neurons; it is also a vasodilator, which helps get oxygen to the brain.

● Anti-inflammatory   ● Mental clarity

Asparagus

Asparagus is a powerful anti-aging vegetable, preventing cell damage in the brain. An important antioxidant found in asparagus, glutathione, may be the foundation for the vegetable's detoxifying effect. Asparagus is high in vitamin B_{12} and folate (B_9), which together promote improved brain functioning, including response speed and cognitive flexibility. Fresh local asparagus available in the spring contains the highest concentration of nutrients.

● Anti-inflammatory   ● Cognitive function

● Brain response time   ● Mental clarity

Avocados

This unique vegetable (some call it a fruit) is more than just a healthy fat replacement. Its high fat content makes it a sort of "nutrient booster" when eaten along with fat-soluble nutrients (carotenoids; vitamins D, E, and K). It also contains folate; vitamins B_5, B_6, and C; oleic acid (a strong anti-inflammatory); and monounsaturated fats, which help lower blood cholesterol.

● Anti-inflammatory   ● Memory

Beets

Beautiful beets are a rich source of folate, a regulator of homo-cysteine levels (helpful in preventing cognitive decline). They contain phytochemicals in their bright red pigment. Researchers have found that drinking beet juice both decreases blood pressure and increases blood flow in the brain, potentially combating the progression of dementia. For a new twist, try freshly grated beets in salads and sandwiches.

● Anti-inflammatory   ● Cognitive function   ● Mental clarity

Broccoli

Due to the strong nutrient profile of broccoli, it has received posi-tive press for years. In addition to containing sulforaphane, a potent antioxidant with nerve-protecting benefits, broccoli is rich in important mind-empowering vitamins A, B_5, C, and E. Broccoli also contains vitamin K, which has been linked with improved cognition in aging.

● Anti-inflammatory   ● Cognitive function   ● Nerve function

Brussels Sprouts

Tasty Brussels sprouts are becoming popular for their vitamin A partner, retinoic acid, which boosts nerve connections and com-bats neurological disorders, including dementia. Also high in vitamins B_6, C, and K; folate; and fiber, this cruciferous vegetable is a brain-boosting dynamo. Brussels sprouts taste best when cut into small pieces and are delicious when cooked with olive oil and garlic, or served raw in salads.

● Anti-inflammatory   ● Cognitive function   ● Nerve function

Carrots

Rich in beta-carotene, vitamins A, B, and folate, carrots are a slam dunk for a healthy mind. Vitamin A and beta-carotene are both strong antioxidants, reducing the risk of cancer as well as memory loss, while vitamins B_6 and B_{12} aid in the regulation of homocysteine levels in the blood; increased levels of this protein by-product are associated with dementia.

• Cognitive function   • Memory

Cauliflower

Unlike many white foods, cauliflower is highly nutritious and loaded with vitamin C and choline-rich fiber. People with higher choline levels have outperformed others on cognitive testing. Cauliflower, a cruciferous vegetable, also contains loads of anti-oxidants and vitamin K, both vitally important for the prevention of Alzheimer's and cardiovascular diseases.

• Anti-inflammatory   • Brain response time   • Cognitive function

Chile Peppers

Capsaicin is the main phytochemical (bioactive plant compound with brain-boosting benefits) found in chile peppers and is responsible for their unique hot taste and many of their health advantages. Other nutrients found in chile peppers are linked to improved cognition, reduced cardiovascular risk, and lowered Alzheimer's risk. These nutrients include vitamins A, B_6, C, and K, and potassium. To help fire up your brain, many chile varieties exist. When dried (cayenne, chili powder), they can add flavor and color to a plethora of dishes.

• Anti-inflammatory   • Concentration
• Cognitive function   • Nerve function

Cucumbers

Belonging to the same family as melons, cucumbers contain a robust phytochemical, fisetin. This antioxidant is effective at protecting the neurons of the brain and can improve memory. It can also decrease inflammation in the body and brain and has a positive effect on brain cells.

• Anti-inflammatory　　• Memory　　• Nerve function

Eggplant

Also called aubergine, eggplant is commonly eaten in Japan and the Mediterranean and Middle Eastern countries. Eggplant contains a strong phytochemical in its skin called nasunin. This potent antioxidant has been shown to protect cell membranes from free radical damage, in turn providing brain protection from Alzheimer's disease. Eggplant is also a good source of dietary fiber, which is associated with lowering the risk of Alzheimer's.

• Anti-inflammatory　　• Cell regeneration　　• Nerve function

Garlic

Affectionately called "a stinking rose," garlic is as healthy as it is fragrant. Garlic, a vegetable bulb, is high in vitamins C and B_6 and in selenium, and has been associated with enhanced memory function and cardiovascular protection through the dilation of blood vessels and control of blood pressure. Fresh garlic contains a wealth of sulfur-containing compounds, which gives it its scent and provides its antioxidant effects. To maximize garlic's nutrient activity, chop it fresh and wait for 5 to 10 minutes before cooking or eating it.

• Anti-inflammatory　　• Cognitive function　　• Memory

Jicama

Sometimes known as the Mexican turnip or potato, jicama adds great crunch and a mild flavor to foods. When combined with the complementary flavors of chili powder, orange juice, and lemon juice, it is powerful food for the brain. Jicama is an excellent source of vitamin C, which can protect your blood vessels from damage that may lead to a stroke, a heart attack, or Alzheimer's disease. It also contains vitamin B_6, which is helpful in the reduction of damaging proteins in the brain.

* Anti-inflammatory   * Cognitive function

Kohlrabi

Raw or cooked, a serving of this cabbage-family vegetable contains more vitamin C than an orange. Much like other cruciferous vegetables, kohlrabi is full of remarkable phytochemicals that reduce inflammation and in turn reduce the risk of developing Alzheimer's disease.

* Anti-Inflammatory   * Cognitive function

Leeks

Related to onions, garlic, and shallots, leeks are an excellent source of antioxidants that fight to protect the cells in the brain. They also contain vitamins A, B_6, C, K, and folate, plus polyphenols, all nutrients that help reduce inflammation and the modifiable risks for Alzheimer's disease.

* Anti-Inflammatory   * Cognitive function   * Cell regeneration

Okra

This ancient Middle Eastern food was traditionally consumed by scholarly students as a "brain food." There is speculation that okra may reduce free radical–induced oxidative stress. Okra pairs well with hot chile peppers or spices such as turmeric and curry.

 • Anti-inflammatory   • Cognitive function

Onions

A close relative to garlic and a member of the allium family, the onion plays a major role as a base seasoning in Mediterranean cuisine. Onions have a positive effect on almost every aspect of brain health: They reduce cardiovascular risk, improve blood pressure, decrease risk of diabetes, decrease homocysteine levels, and have prebiotic functions. Incorporating onions daily into your mind-nourishing eating plan is a recipe for brain health.

 • Anti-inflammatory   • Cognitive function   • Memory

Potatoes

The potent potato is frequently underestimated and takes a bad rap for the unhealthy preparation methods and toppings added to it. Promising studies reveal that the antioxidant properties in potatoes can improve memory deficit in individuals with cognitive loss. Vitamins B_6 and C, potassium, and fiber may help sharpen mental focus and avoid long-term cognitive decline. In an effort to keep your brain healthy, consume the versatile potato—skin and all to provide the protection you need.

 • Anti-inflammatory   • Concentration
 • Cognitive function   • Memory

Pumpkins

Roasted, baked, boiled, or dried, pumpkins bring home the brain boost needed to lessen your risk of Alzheimer's disease. The B-vitamin content may raise cognitive-skill test scores, and the vitamins A and C from this bright orange vegetable protect against cardiovascular disease and help with memory and learning new mental skills.

- Anti-inflammatory
- Concentration
- Nerve function
- Cognitive function
- Memory

Red Bell Peppers

Although all bell peppers have great nutritional qualities for a healthy brain, the red variety actually provides more vitamin C than its green, yellow, or orange counterparts, and more than even citrus fruit. Along with vitamin A, a network of antioxidants support the immune system and reduce inflammation and cell damage in the brain. Vitamins B_6, C, E, and K, plus potassium and folate, add to the total mind-health package of this flavorful vegetable.

- Anti-inflammatory
- Cognitive function
- Nerve function

Red Cabbage

Red cabbage has a specific compound that activates a good protein responsible for getting rid of bad tau proteins formed in the brain. Tau proteins act as a transport system for nutrients throughout the brain, and when altered become tangled and slowly degrade. These tangled proteins are highly prominent in the brains of Alzheimer's patients. Red cabbage provides a significant brain boost due to its protective red pigments.

- Anti-inflammatory
- Concentration
- Mental clarity
- Cognitive function
- Memory

Shiitake Mushrooms

Chinese culture has embraced the shiitake mushroom for medicinal purposes for more than 6,000 years. These flavorful fungi can now be purchased in most grocery stores in the produce aisle or at farmers' markets. They are a good source of vitamin B_5, selenium, and antioxidants, which play crucial roles in brain health. Mushrooms have been linked to immune system protection, inflammation protection, and enhancement of nerve growth in the brain.

- Anti-inflammatory
- Nerve function
- Nerve growth

Sweet Potatoes

The anti-inflammation effect of sweet potatoes is extremely proficient at protecting brain tissue. This food is high in beta-carotene; vitamins A, B complex, C, and E; and phytochemicals, specifically the antioxidant anthocyanin. This combination of powerful nutrients may boost the brain's learning skills, enhance the ability to focus, and decrease risk of Alzheimer's by reducing cell damage in the brain. For more information on this powerful food, see the next page.

- Anti-inflammatory
- Cognitive function
- Nerve function
- Brain response time
- Concentration

Sweet Potatoes

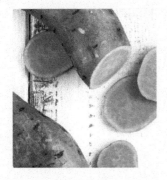

Baked, mashed, roasted, or boiled—no matter how you cook them, sweet potatoes are sure to nourish and protect your brain. Sweet potatoes are one of the oldest vegetables known to humans.

- This orange-fleshed root veggie is one of the best sources of vitamin A and beta-carotene in the US food supply.
- Supplying fiber and a high concentration of other nutrients, the sweet potato has shown promise as a food to help reduce the incidence of Alzheimer's disease.
- Sweet potatoes are a staple for many countries, including Japan, which boasts of having a low rate of Alzheimer's.
- The beautiful sweet potato is not always orange on the inside. There is another variety that is purple-fleshed and has a different set of phytochemicals, including the brain powerhouse anthocyanin. Regardless of the color, though, sweet potatoes are a great source of a wide variety of vitamins and antioxidants.

This age-old vegetable is having a resurgence as a popular replacement for fried and baked potatoes on restaurant menus. Adding sweet potatoes to the brain-healthy diet a couple of times a week is easy: Just replace them in any recipe calling for another root vegetable, or use them in casseroles or as a side dish for any meal of the day.

Tomatoes

Tomatoes are a brain-health force, rich in all four of the major carotenoids, antioxidants (beta-carotene, vitamins A and C), vitamin B_5, and potassium. The antioxidants help prevent harmful by-products in the body from forming and damaging the cells. Additionally, the potassium found in tomatoes is important for nerve and muscle function.

* Cognitive function   * Memory   * Nerve function

Winter Squash

Winter squash can help keep your brain healthy. While butternut, delicata, Hubbard, spaghetti, and kabocha squashes are all packed with nutrients, acorn squash is the gray-matter powerhouse. Nutrients in winter squash that contribute to improved cognition, learning skills, and decreased cell damage in the brain include vitamins A, B_6, C, and K; folate; and potassium, and fiber.

* Anti-inflammatory   * Concentration   * Nerve function
* Cognitive function   * Memory

Yams

Sometimes confused with sweet potatoes, the yam is a sweet root tuber of varying sizes and colors—from pink to tan to purple. Touted as a "superfood" with multiple health benefits, yams help with Alzheimer's prevention through their alphabet of vitamins (A, B, C, E, and K) and abundance of antioxidants, fiber, and magnesium. The darker colors have the biggest array of brain-power nutrients.

- Anti-inflammatory
- Concentration
- Nerve function
- Cognitive function
- Memory

Zucchini

Sweet and delicate enough to be eaten raw or cooked, zucchini is a summertime favorite, yet it is available in most supermarkets year around. Because of its high water content, this vegetable has a great nutrient-to-calorie ratio (high nutrients, low calories) and provides many of the nutrients important for brain health. Folate, along with vitamins A and C, helps protect the cells in the heart and brain from damage that may lead to Alzheimer's and cardiovascular disease.

- Anti-inflammatory
- Cognitive function

FRUIT

Apricots

These small orange-colored fruits have a dense concentration of antioxidants to help reduce free radicals in the body and brain, and flavonoids to slow cognitive decline. They are also rich in fiber and carotenoids, which decrease cardiovascular risk.

• Anti-inflammatory   • Cognitive function   • Memory

Berries

Blueberries. Cranberries. Blackberries. Raspberries. Strawberries. They are all delicious and good for your brain. Not only do they lower blood pressure and cholesterol and benefit the cardiovascular system, berries have also been shown to increase memory and cognition. Berries are full of flavonoids, antioxidants, and phytonutrients. Studies done on individuals with mild cognitive impairment showed berries can increase memory and word recognition. For more information on this powerful brain food, see the next page.

• Anti-inflammatory   • Cognitive function   • Memory

Cherries

Whether sweet or tart, cherries promote brain health. Filled with the phytochemical anthocyanin, and the antioxidants from anthocyanin and vitamin C, cherries help the body's cells defend themselves against oxidative damage.

• Anti-inflammatory   • Memory
• Cognitive function   • Sleep enhancement

Berries

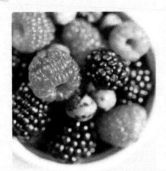

While blueberries have grabbed most of the limelight, this entire category of fruit deserves the title "superfood." Some of the most compelling evidence for berries includes the brain-health connection.

- Simply put, berries provide brain protection and help ward off dementia and Alzheimer's disease.

The reason for this is a bit complicated and is associated with their phytochemical composition—anthocyanins, catechins, quercetins, kaempferols, and tannins. These antioxidant and anti-inflammatory compounds work together to inhibit brain aging and the progression of neurodegenerative disorders.

- There is growing interest in the potential of the natural polyphenols in berries to improve memory, learning, and general cognitive abilities. One such polyphenol found in blueberries is resveratrol, which is also prominent in red wine.

Eating a small portion of berries every day is not excessive. However, they are a seasonal food, typically available from April to October. During the winter months, frozen berries provide a good option. Try using them at least several times a week in smoothies, with whole-grain cereals, or as a snack.

Citrus

In the mid-1700s, citrus fruit was used to prevent and cure scurvy in the British navy; today it is found in abundance in our supermarkets. Citrus has high anti-inflammatory properties, flavonoids, phytonutrients, and many antioxidants (most prominently vitamin C). Oranges, grapefruit, lemons, and limes are excellent additions to any diet, especially when taking Alzheimer's prevention into consideration.

• Anti-inflammatory   • Cognitive function

Grapes

One of the oldest fruits known to humankind, grapes—both red and purple—are an excellent food for an Alzheimer's prevention diet. They are rich in antioxidants, as well as vitamins B_6, C, and K; flavonoids (a strong anti-inflammatory); phytonutrients; and carotenoids. Many of the nutrients including a hearty dose of resveratrol, are contained in the skin of the dark-colored fruit. Because of their high fiber content, grapes are also excellent for overall health.

• Anti-inflammatory   • Brain response time   • Cell regeneration

Mangos

Whether blended in a smoothie, added to a salsa, or just eaten plain, mangos are an excellent choice for a well-rounded fruit. They are known to help decrease the risk of many diseases, not the least of which is cognitive decline. This is the result of the strong antioxidants they have (flavonoids and vitamins B_6, C, and E). For an added brain boost, they contain lots of fiber and vitamin A.

• Anti-inflammatory   • Brain response time   • Mental clarity

Melons

Melons, in particular honeydews and bitter melons, are packed full of B vitamins, vitamin C, and phytochemicals that play a large role in brain health. Studies have shown the polyphenol antioxidants in melons may have a protective effect on the brain. Melons make a sweet addition to any meal or snack.

● Anti-inflammatory   ● Cognitive function

Plantains

Plantains are a staple in the cuisine of many countries and are associated with increased longevity and decreased risk of Alzheimer's disease. Often prepared in a similar fashion to potatoes, plantains are an interesting choice for replacing a carbohydrate in a meal. They are high in fiber, contain more vitamin A and C than bananas, and are rich in potassium and vitamin B_6, all connected with improved memory and decreased damage caused by free radicals in brain cells.

● Anti-inflammatory   ● Cognitive function   ● Memory

Plums

The mighty plum is a great fruit choice for the brain, as it is loaded with fiber, potassium, and vitamins C and K. The Kakadu plum, native to Australia, has received especially high praise for its antioxidant profile, which is thought to reduce toxic beta-amyloid proteins in the brains of individuals with Alzheimer's disease. Watch for forthcoming research on this nutritionally-potent fruit.

● Anti-inflammatory   ● Cognitive function

Pomegranates

Pomegranates are a potent fruit with a diverse nutritional profile. The juice of the pomegranate contains powerful antioxidants, including vitamins C and E, which protect brain cells from oxidation and cognitive decline. The fruit is also high in anthocyanin, the red pigment that protects the body against neurological damage and atherosclerosis in large blood vessels.

- Anti-inflammatory
- Cognitive function
- Memory
- Nerve function

LEGUMES

Beans

Many cultures with high life expectancy and low incidence of Alzheimer's disease, such as the Japanese and Mediterranean cultures, eat beans as a staple in their food supplies. Dried beans, an inexpensive, protein-rich legume, are a great source of fiber, folate, magnesium, and potassium—all nutrients that slow cognitive decline. Colored beans possess greater antioxidant properties than white beans. Beans also contain choline, a vitamin-like compound essential for brain development, which may potentially improve communication in the brain and prevent age-related memory loss.

- Anti-inflammatory
- Brain response time
- Memory
- Nerve growth

Black-Eyed Peas

Fiber and phytochemicals in black-eyed peas can reduce the risk of cardiovascular disease and inflammation in the body and brain. Black-eyed peas are packed with many other important nutrients, including folate, magnesium, and iron, a potent brain-health combo. These earthy-tasting legumes pair marvelously with the brain-healthy foods parsley and lemon juice.

- Anti-inflammatory
- Cognitive function
- Memory

Garbanzo Beans (Chickpeas)

Garbanzos, or chickpeas, were first cultivated in the Middle East and eventually worked their way into diets across the globe. Garbanzo beans are extremely high in fiber and invaluable in digestive and colon health. They are also rich in antioxidants (vitamins C and E), phytonutrients (flavonoids), folate, and potassium, all of which make this legume a slam-dunk brain food. For more information on this powerful brain food, see the next page.

• Anti-inflammatory   • Cognitive function

• Cell regeneration   • Memory

Lentils

These versatile legumes are easy to include in many dishes due to their complementary flavor and texture. Studies conducted over several decades have suggested that increasing consumption of plant foods like lentils decreases the risk of obesity, diabetes, heart disease, and overall mortality. Lentils provide B vitamins, which are specifically beneficial to lower homocysteine levels in the brain; a high level is linked to increased risk for Alzheimer's disease.

• Anti-inflammatory   • Cognitive function   • Memory

Mung Beans

This ancient bean from Asia has been eaten for many centuries and possesses great promise as an anti-Alzheimer's superfood. The mung bean is loaded with antioxidants and phytochemicals, which can help reduce damaging oxidation in the brain, providing brain protection. Mung beans are highly versatile and can be eaten cooked or sprouted.

• Anti-inflammatory   • Cognitive function

A CLOSER LOOK

Garbanzo Beans

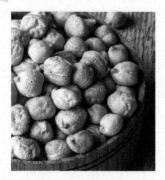

Garbanzo beans, also known as chick-peas, lead the legume category for their brain-protection capabilities. The consumption of legumes improves cognition and prevents damage from oxidation in the body and brain.

- The garbanzo bean's outer seed coat has concentrated mind-nourishing flavonoids, including quercetin, kaempferol, and myricetin, while the interior is rich in ferulic, chlorogenic, caffeic, and vanillic acids. All of these phytochemicals function as antioxidants.
- Studies suggest the garbanzo's phytochemicals may decrease chronic inflammation and increase self-destruction of damaged brain cells.
- Garbanzo beans are an excellent source of the healthy-brain nutrients folate and fiber.
- Research suggests that diets that include beans reduce low-density lipoprotein cholesterol, favorably affect risk factors for metabolic syndrome, and reduce risk of heart disease and diabetes. These risk factors are consistent with the modifiable risks for development of Alzheimer's disease.

Eat garbanzos and other legumes in ½-cup servings at least three or four times per week to lower the risk of Alzheimer's disease. Garbanzos can be used in main dishes, soups, salads, as sides, and even as a fat replacement in baking.

Peanuts

An allergen to some, peanuts may help nourish and protect the brains of others. They are a great source of vitamin E, which functions as an antioxidant and protects nerve membranes. Peanuts are also an excellent source of B vitamins, especially niacin; all of the B vitamins have positive attributes for brain health.

• Anti-inflammatory   • Cognitive function   • Nerve function

Soybeans

Found in many products, soybeans are a very diverse protein source with a high concentration of many nutrients. They help slow cognitive decline and improve overall brain function with their content of folate, vitamin K, calcium, riboflavin, and flavonoids. They are an excellent source of fiber, contain a variety of other essential vitamins and minerals, and are fun to eat out of the shell as edamame.

• Anti-inflammatory   • Cognitive function

WHOLE GRAINS

Amaranth

This ancient grain is gaining popularity due to its wide array of nutrients and many health benefits. Amaranth, a gluten-free whole grain, contains heart-healthy oleic fatty acids and polyphenols (plant compounds with antioxidant and anti-inflammatory effects). These nutrients help protect the brain and aid in the repair of damaged brain cells. Amaranth can be popped like popcorn, or eaten as a hot cereal for breakfast or as a savory side dish combined with almost any spice or herb from this guide.

- Anti-inflammatory
- Cognitive function

Barley

The B-vitamin content of barley, including folate, B_6, and B_{12}, makes it a "grain for your brain." The consumption of B-vitamin-rich foods has been linked to lowered homocysteine levels in the blood, causing memory-boosting effects and lessened cognitive decline. Additionally, the high fiber in this whole grain contributes to improved blood sugar regulation and lowered cardiovascular risk, resulting in lowered Alzheimer's risk.

- Cognitive function
- Memory

Brown Rice

The Mediterranean and MIND diets both support the use of whole grains versus refined carbohydrates for the prevention of Alzheimer's disease. Brown rice is one such whole grain, and studies show substituting brown rice for white rice can reduce the incidence of type 2 diabetes, which is linked to increased Alzheimer's risk. Brown rice has antioxidative compounds, is rich in fiber and selenium, and is a good choice for nourishment of the mind.

• Cognitive function   • Memory

Buckwheat

Despite its name, this whole grain is a seed, not a wheat, which also means it is gluten-free. Buckwheat is higher in protein than other grains and has a nutritional profile that demonstrates brain-health potential. It is high in magnesium, folate, fiber, and selenium. Buckwheat contains many brain-defending phytochemicals. One in particular, rutin, works together with vitamin C to form a strong antioxidant, which protects brain cells from damage.

• Anti-inflammatory   • Cognitive function

Bulgur

Packed with insoluble fiber, bulgur has qualities to help reduce cholesterol, regulate blood sugars, and potentially reduce the risk of Alzheimer's disease. This Middle Eastern staple complements a variety of herbs, spices, and other foods. Bulgur is a good source of potassium, which supports the brain's memory function. It is also a slowly absorbed source of glucose for the brain.

• Cognitive function   • Memory

Farro

An ancient Egyptian grain used in Italian cooking for centuries, farro is an excellent alternative to pasta or rice. This tiny nourishing whole grain is packed with several important minerals. One mineral vital to brain health is magnesium. Inadequate magnesium intake can lead to elevated inflammatory markers in the body, increased heart disease, diabetes, and Alzheimer's risk. Magnesium is also important to promote adequate sleep.

- Anti-inflammatory
- Cognitive function
- Nerve function
- Sleep enhancement

Millet

This gluten-free grain is often overlooked, but it is an excellent option for any diet, especially for brain-health benefits. It is high in both protein and fiber, as well as magnesium, all of which are important nutrients with regard to Alzheimer's prevention. Additionally, millet is an excellent source of many B vitamins and is one of the best grain sources of antioxidants.

- Anti-inflammatory
- Cognitive function
- Nerve function

Oats

More than just a breakfast cereal, oats provide a brain boost any time of the day. Oats defend your heart and brain with their high levels of soluble fiber (which reduces cholesterol and stabilizes blood sugars) and B vitamins. This nourishing whole grain also contains zinc and potassium—nutrients vital to brain development and helpful for full-capacity brain function. Benefits are consistent regardless of the type of oats eaten (quick, old-fashioned, steel-cut).

- Cognitive function
- Memory

Spelt

An ancient grain, spelt is part of the wheat, rye, and barley family. Spelt is light in texture, with a slightly nutty flavor. Rich in B vitamins, magnesium, zinc, iron, and manganese, it may be one of the healthiest grains for your brain. In addition to its high fiber content, it also has twice as much vitamin K as wheat. Vitamin K plays an important role in the nervous system and brain cell communication.

• Anti-inflammatory   • Cognitive function   • Nerve function

Wheat Germ

This is the nutrient-rich powerhouse part of the wheat kernel and is a promising brain-enhancing food. Wheat germ is a good source of vitamin E. When derived from food versus supplementation, this powerful antioxidant vitamin has been linked to a decreased risk of Alzheimer's disease in some studies. Wheat germ is also high in B vitamins, zinc, and magnesium, which are important nutrients in overall brain health.

• Anti-inflammatory   • Memory

NUTS AND SEEDS

Almonds

For years almonds have been appreciated for their monounsaturated fat content and their ability to decrease blood cholesterol levels and the risk of heart disease. Today, researchers are taking a closer look at the excellent cognitive contributions in this little nut—antioxidants (vitamin E), vitamins, and minerals (such as magnesium and potassium).

• Anti-inflammatory   • Cognitive function

Chia Seeds

These tiny, tasteless seeds are full of selenium, a nutrient vital for proper brain communication. Chia seeds also contain omega-3 alpha-linolenic (ALA) fatty acids, which studies show reduce age-related mental decline. As a bonus, chia seeds are loaded with antioxidants to reduce cell damage and inflammation in the brain.

• Anti-inflammatory   • Cognitive function   • Memory

Flaxseeds

Known for reducing the risk of some cancers, heart disease, stroke, diabetes, and (most recently) Alzheimer's, flaxseed has been pegged as one of the most beneficial plant foods. Flax is dense with omega-3 fatty acids, which are associated with slowing memory decline. It also contains many vitamins and nutrients such as iron, calcium, potassium, magnesium, folate, and thiamine, as well as several antioxidants and phytonutrients.

• Anti-inflammatory   • Cognitive function   • Memory

Hazelnuts

Sometimes called filberts, these tree nuts are an energy-dense food due to their high content of monounsaturated fats, which decrease cholesterol, the risk of heart disease, and the risk of Alzheimer's disease. In addition to their heart-healthy benefits, hazelnuts are packed full of antioxidants like vitamin A, and phytochemicals such as vitamin E, flavonoids, and carotenoids—all powerful brain-positive compounds.

• Anti-inflammatory   • Cognitive function

Pecans

This nut is one of the richest sources of antioxidants, vitamin A, B vitamins, calcium, potassium, magnesium, and choline. With a winning nutrient combination such as that, it is no wonder pecans are thought to be protective for the heart and the brain. They are also high in omega-3 fatty acids, which are important for cognition preservation.

• Anti-inflammatory   • Cognitive function   • Memory

Pistachios

These delicious green nuts are a mainstay in the Mediterranean diet. Besides fiber, potassium, and folate, they are also known for containing resveratrol, the same brain-powerful phytonutrient found in red wine. Pistachios have high levels of essential fatty acids and vitamin E to help prevent inflammation in the brain.

• Anti-inflammatory   • Cognitive function   • Memory

Pumpkin Seeds

Yum! These crunchy little nuggets are full of many vitamins and nutrients that benefit both body and brain. They contain large amounts of the antioxidant vitamin E in many forms, as well as the phytonutrient lignin, which has been linked to helping prolong survival in cancer patients. Additionally, pumpkin seeds contain vitamin C, niacin, folate, and potassium, which help protect the brain from damage due to Alzheimer's.

• Anti-inflammatory   • Memory

Walnuts

This tasty nut touts the highest amount of alpha-linolenic acid (ALA) in its class. ALA is a plant-based omega-3 essential fatty acid that enhances cognition. Walnuts contain high levels of polyphenols, naturally occurring compounds in foods linked to preserving cognition and protecting against dementia. Studies point to the combination of antioxidants and ALA to protect brain cells and DNA from oxidation and inflammation. Besides walnuts, other good sources of ALA are flaxseeds, canola oil, dairy products, and eggs. For more information on this powerful brain food, see A Closer Look (page 87).

• Anti-inflammatory   • Cognitive function   • Memory

OILS

Coconut Oil

This solid oil is full of saturated, monounsaturated, and polyunsaturated fatty acids, but, most pertinent to Alzheimer's studies, the majority of the fats are medium-chain triglycerides. These triglycerides can easily be converted into ketones, which in turn become an energy source for the brain. This process occurs due to their ability to passively enter the bloodstream without using transport channels. Studies are underway and conclusive research is needed to determine the efficacy of coconut oil as a main fat and calorie source for Alzheimer's disease prevention. Another positive in the brain-health court is that coconut oil contains vitamin E, which has been linked with delayed memory loss.

• Cognitive function   • Memory

Extra-Virgin Olive Oil

For years, olive oil has been known for its cardiovascular, blood cholesterol, and digestive health benefits. Studies have shown that, in particular, extra-virgin olive oil (EVOO) has a stronger concentration of phytonutrients than regular olive oil. It also has more oleic acid (monounsaturated fat), which has strong anti-inflammatory properties. One of the foundations of the brain-healthy Mediterranean diet, EVOO has been implicated in the removal of beta-amyloid proteins in the brain, which could be part of the reason why countries with a very high intake of this nutritious oil have lower rates of Alzheimer's disease.

• Anti-inflammatory   • Memory
• Cognitive function   • Nerve function

Walnuts

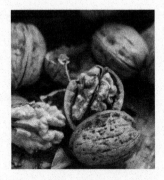

Walnuts are tree nuts that have been cultivated for thousands of years. There are several different varieties, with black walnuts being the most common type found in the United States.

- Walnuts are a rich source of plant-based omega-3 fatty acids and are particularly high in one type called alpha-linolenic acid, or ALA. Walnuts are one of the most significant sources of ALA, an essential fatty acid. The word *essential* here means your body cannot synthesize it, so it has to be eaten in the diet. Research links a high intake of omega-3s to a reduction in risk for cognitive decline. Theories about why omega-3s might influence dementia risk include their anti-inflammatory effects and their support and protection of nerve cell membranes.
- Other nutrients found in abundance in the delicious, nutritious walnut include folate, vitamin B_6, vitamin E, and fiber—all influential in nourishing the brain.

Roast walnuts and toss them into salads or with whole grains. Grind them to make dips and spreads. Pair them with leafy greens, cinnamon, and other brain-healthy foods.

PROTEIN

Eggs

Eggs were a demonized food for decades, but recent research points toward the many benefits of more than just the white part of this protein-packed food. Egg yolks contain the strong antioxidant vitamin E and the nutrient choline. Both are essential for brain development and potentially instrumental in the prevention of age-related memory loss. Eggs also have other important nutrients, including vitamins B and D and selenium. Farm-fresh and omega 3–enriched eggs wield the biggest nutritional impact.

- Anti-inflammatory
- Brain response time
- Concentration
- Memory
- Nerve growth

Fish

In the United States, the average person eats about 15 pounds of fish per year. By contrast, people in Japan and countries of the Mediterranean consume four to five times this amount, and their incidence of Alzheimer's is lower and their life expectancy is higher. Brain health is dependent upon omega-3 fatty acids and vitamin D, both of which are prominent in fatty fish. For more information on this powerful brain food, see the next page.

- Anti-inflammatory
- Cognitive function
- Concentration
- Nerve function
- Nerve growth
- Memory
- Sleep enhancement

Fish

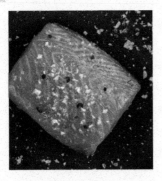

Fatty fish is the world's best source of omega-3 fatty acids and the best dietary source of vitamin D, an essential nutrient deficient in over 40 percent of the US population. Both nutrients are important in the prevention of heart attack, stroke, and Alzheimer's disease and are crucial for brain development and to reduce brain shrinkage and function as we age.

The following fish have more than 5 percent fat by weight and are ranked from highest to lowest by omega-3 fatty acid composition:

- Mackerel
- Lake trout
- Herring
- Wild salmon
- Carp/chub
- American shad
- Sardines

- Chilean sea bass
- Sablefish/black cod
- Whitefish
- Butterfish/pompano
- Tuna
- Anchovies
- Eel

Fish with high mercury contamination, such as Chilean king mackerel, swordfish, shark, marlin, sablefish, Chilean sea bass, and some varieties of tuna, should be eaten in limited quantities (avoid if pregnant, may become pregnant, or breastfeeding).

Eat 3 to 4 ounces of fatty fish at least three times per week. Taking fish oil supplements does not show the same positive results for cognition.

Tofu

Epidemiological studies observed that populations that consume greater amounts of soy have, in general, lower rates of age-related mental disorders. Although soy consumption was possibly linked with increased dementia in one study in the early 2000s, the overall health benefits outweigh the risks. Tofu and other soy foods contain phytonutrients that protect the heart and brain and may improve memory and cognition.

- Cognitive function
- Memory
- Nerve function

FERMENTED FOODS

Apple Cider Vinegar

While its full effects on brain health are still being researched, apple cider vinegar has been used as a medical remedy for centuries. Friendly bacteria (probiotics) and antioxidants are thought to be the mechanism for reducing health risks. This fermented vinegar has shown promise in improving insulin sensitivity and cardiovascular risk, although human studies are still needed.

• Anti-inflammatory

Craft Beer

Rich in flavonoids (a phytochemical plant compound), B vitamins, probiotics, and (often) brain-enriching additions such as herbs and spices, craft beer may just be the new liquid refreshment for brain health. Though caution should be used to avoid overconsumption, one beer per day for women and two for men may prove to have brain-protective effects through a reduction of cardiovascular risks and inflammation.

• Anti-inflammatory   • Cognitive function

Kefir

This fermented milk drink contains high levels of brain-enriching vitamin B_{12} and folate and is filled with probiotics. Certain strains of bacteria in kefir have been linked to improved learning and memory. The probiotics also play a role in reducing inflammation, which lowers Alzheimer's risk.

• Anti-inflammatory   • Cognitive function   • Memory

Miso

Many Asian cultures have lower incidence of Alzheimer's disease. Miso has been an important part of these cultures for centuries. Miso is a pasty food composed primarily of fermented soybeans and is often made into soup. It is a very good source of manganese and vitamin K, both important for brain function. Soybeans are also one of the richest sources of phytochemicals (isoflavones), which may mimic the role of estrogen in the brain.

• Cognitive function   • Nerve function

Red Wine

There have been many studies linking moderate daily consumption of red wine to a slowed progression of Alzheimer's disease. Most of these studies point to the phytochemical resveratrol in red wine as the protective agent that restores healthy-brain components and reduces brain inflammation. For more information on this powerful brain food, see the next page.

• Anti-inflammatory   • Cognitive function   • Memory

Sauerkraut

Fermented cabbage in the form of fresh sauerkraut is rich in vitamins B, C, and K. In fact, the fermentation process increases the availability of these vitamins and makes the sauerkraut even more nutritious than its raw, unfermented form. This is good news for brain health, as in addition, sauerkraut is rich in probiotics, antioxidants, fiber, folate, potassium, and magnesium, which are all important in improving cognition.

• Anti-inflammatory   • Concentration
• Cognitive function   • Mental clarity

Red Wine

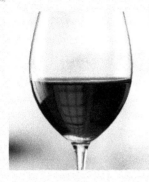

What are the secrets behind red wine and a healthy brain?

- Red wine is particularly high in the phytochemical resveratrol, a polyphenol found in grape skins and touted as a possible preventive compound for Alzheimer's disease, cancer, diabetes, and many other conditions. The amount of resveratrol in wine depends on the type of red grape used and the region in which it is grown. Generally there is more of this phytochemical in the grapes grown in cooler climates. Pinot Noir, Malbec, Cannonau, and Grenache wines have the highest content of resveratrol.

- New research on the effects of resveratrol for Alzheimer's disease prevention suggests it may actually slow the progression of the disease by protecting nerve cells from damage and fighting plaque buildup in the brain.

How does this research translate into recommendations? The American Heart Association recommends drinking in moderation for heart health, which amounts to an average of one to two drinks per day for men, and one drink per day for women. Following these recommendations may have the added benefit of preventing Alzheimer's disease.

Yogurt

Live-culture yogurt with probiotics has been shown to improve cognition and reduce anxiety. Some studies suggest that the GI tract microbiome (the large family of good bacteria in the gut) in Alzheimer's patients is altered and that probiotics improve learning through the gut's influence on neurological function. Plain yogurt, both Greek and regular, are great choices.

- Brain response time
- Memory
- Cognitive function
- Sleep enhancement

OTHER

Coffee

Fortunately for java fans, coffee consumption (without added cream and sugar) has been linked to up to 65 percent lowered incidence of Alzheimer's disease. Beyond the caffeine, coffee's hearty dose of antioxidants, positive anti-inflammatory action, and ability to reduce insulin resistance have all been cited for their positive effects on the brain. Since coffee is a stimulant, it is not for everyone and can interrupt sleep, especially if consumed later in the day.

• Anti-inflammatory   • Cognitive function   • Concentration

Green Tea

The antioxidants from the flavonoids and catechin phytochemical groups present in green tea may help catapult it to the top of the mind-healthy food list. Studies have revealed that individuals who drink more green tea show improved mental focus, better memory, heightened brain activity, and the creation of new neurons in the brain. Green tea provides a great opportunity for the addition of other brain-healthy spices, herbs, and fruits. For more information on this powerful brain food, see A Closer Look (page 97).

• Anti-inflammatory   • Concentration   • Nerve growth

• Cognitive function   • Nerve function

Seaweed

This powerful antioxidant food is a staple of the Japanese diet. Complex nutritious compounds (sulfated polysaccharides) found in seaweed have been shown to reverse oxidative damage to brain and nerve cells. A chemical called homotaurine is also found in seaweed and has been linked to reducing brain toxins and interfering with the formation of the plaques in the brain that contribute to Alzheimer's disease. Homotaurines are found only in certain types of seaweed, and not in supplements.

● Anti-Inflammatory   ● Cognitive function   ● Memory

Green Tea

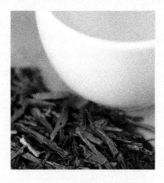

What makes green tea the healthiest beverage for your brain? Is it the anti-oxidants, the caffeine, or the amino acids? Researchers believe it might be all of these things . . . and maybe more.

- Powerful antioxidants in green tea have been linked to a reduction in damage from free radicals, which are in part responsible for aging and deterioration in the brain.
- The caffeine in green tea blocks bad nerve communicators and increases the concentration of good connections. This in turn leads to improvements in brain function, reaction time, and memory.
- An important amino acid, L-theanine, works with the caffeine in green tea to improve brain productivity.

Collectively, these somewhat complicated reactions in the brain help reduce your risk of developing Alzheimer's disease.

Drinking at least one cup of green tea (iced or hot) per day will add to your arsenal of brain protection. Remember, the highest quality teas are loose leaf. You can add extra brain-nourishing power to your green tea by adding other herbs and spices from this guidebook—try a new one each day.

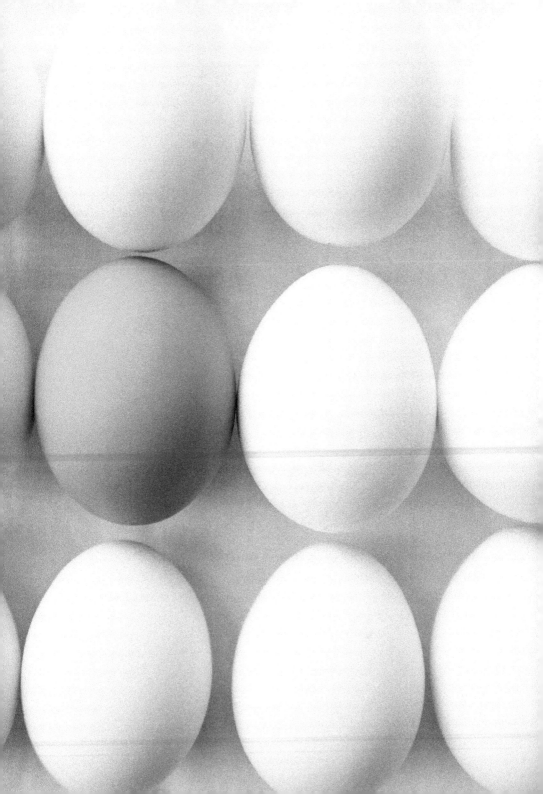

Chapter 4
The Meal Plans

This chapter is where we turn information into action. The sample meal pattern and meal plans presented here take into account the dietary guidance that we covered in chapter 2 and call for a variety of the brain foods we profiled in chapter 3.

To help nourish and protect the brain, the following general guidelines are recommended:

- Don't rush your meals.
- Eat meals with family and friends whenever possible.
- Drink at least 8 ounces of water with every meal and in between meals, too.
- Avoid deep-fried foods.

- Use extra-virgin olive oil (EVOO) as the fat of choice in sautéing and pan-frying; vinaigrettes and sauces; pesto, hummus, and other spreads; and as a replacement for butter or margarine in and on foods such as toast and vegetables.
- Limit high-fat meats, butter, margarine, mayonnaise, and cream, and other high-fat foods.
- Use lean cuts of meat in small portions (less than 5 ounces) a couple of times per week, mainly as a flavoring or condiment in cooking.
- Limit sugar, sweets, pastries, desserts, and sugary drinks to a couple of times per week.
- Use salt in moderation—try new spices and herbs instead.
- Consume protein in the breakfast meal, and evenly distribute protein amounts throughout the day.
- Eat whole fruit versus juice, and limit fruit juices to 4 ounces, three or fewer times per week.
- If you choose to drink alcohol, drink in moderation— one drink for women and two for men, daily.

It may be helpful to use this plate as a visual example to plan your meals using the food categories in this guide:

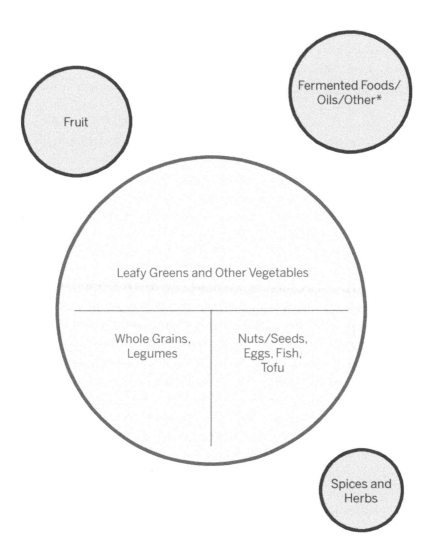

Other foods include coffee, green tea, and seaweed

Sample Meal Pattern

For many, it is overwhelming to think about preparing multiple meals each day. We encourage you to think in terms of meal patterns, or the categories or elements of a meal that you can put together to make up a brain-friendly plate. When you plan for meals at home, thinking in terms of a meal pattern can be helpful. Using the plate diagram as a guide, here is a sample meal pattern for breakfast, lunch, and dinner, plus two optional snacks for any given day. Consider including fermented foods in at least one of these meals or snack times.

Breakfast

- ½ cup or 1 small piece of fruit
- ½ cup hot whole-grain cereal or 1 cup cold cereal or 1 to 2 slices whole-grain bread or ½ cup starchy vegetable or legumes
- 2 ounces protein or ½ to 1 cup dairy (or ¼ of the plate)
- 1 cup coffee or green tea

OPTIONAL: 1 to 2 cups leafy greens or other vegetables

Lunch

- ½ cup or 1 small piece fruit
- 2 cups raw or 1 cup cooked vegetables/leafy greens (or ½ of the plate)
- ½ cup whole grain or 1 to 2 slices whole-grain bread or ½ cup starchy vegetable or legumes
- 3 to 4 ounces protein (or ¼ of the plate)

Dinner

- ½ cup or 1 small piece fruit
- 2 cups raw or 1 cup cooked vegetables/leafy greens (or ½ of the plate)
- ½ cup whole grain or 1 to 2 slices whole-grain bread or ½ cup starchy vegetable or legumes
- 3 to 4 ounces protein (or ¼ of the plate)

OPTIONAL: 1 (6-ounce) glass red wine or 1 (12-ounce) glass craft beer, or 1 cup tea or hot chocolate (made with cacao)

Optional Snack (once or twice daily)

- ½ cup fruit or vegetable
- 1 to 2 ounces protein

Two Weeks of Meal Plans

We have written a two week meal plan, structured to provide the proper number of servings from each food group, as recommended in chapter 2. Each of the brain-healthy foods in the book is incorporated in the meal plan at least once. We made an effort to include the names of recipes that will be easy for you to find online.

Meal planning takes a little work and creativity, but once you get into the habit, you will discover it is worth the effort. Remember, there is no right or wrong way to plan meals. The best advice is to incorporate brain-nourishing foods into every meal, try new things, and mix and match foods that work for you and your family. Having written meal plans for clients over the course of many years, we know they can be difficult to implement to the letter. With that in mind, recognize that you will probably not follow this exactly, and that's okay. Your overall commitment to changing your diet is more important than sticking strictly to this meal plan. Don't be hard on yourself. If you don't eat a single food profiled in this book for three days in a row, accept it and move on. The next day, treat yourself to a mug of green tea and munch on a handful of walnuts when you feel like snacking. Slow change is better than no change at all.

As mentioned previously, fresh, in-season, and organic foods often provide the highest nutrient content and lowest risk of contaminants. However, it is better to eat a wide variety of the foods profiled in this guide in any form rather than bypass them because you cannot afford, or do not have access to, organics. Turn to page 164 to see lists of produce that carry the relative highest and lowest pesticide loads, which can influence whether or not you buy organic varieties. As always, be sure to wash all fresh foods carefully before consuming them.

Simplify Your Menu Prep

There's nothing like a home-cooked meal, and there are some steps you can take to ease the time and stress that sometimes come with the thought of preparing a meal after a difficult or long day at work. Chopping an onion or carrot for your dinner preparation? Chop one or two extra, and store them to use for meals you plan to make later in the week. Or do as much ahead-of-time preparation on the weekends as you can. By chopping and storing vegetables and portioning out your proteins ahead of time, your actual meal prep during the week is only about cooking—and eating—the delicious food.

Other time-saving techniques include preparing double recipes of soups and stews in a slow cooker. The leftovers make for another delicious meal. Likewise, who has time to cook a healthy breakfast every morning? An egg bake or oatmeal can be made in quantity at the beginning of the week and eaten throughout the week. Sauces like marinara, pesto, and chimichurri can be purchased or made ahead of time as well, and will store safely in the refrigerator for a couple of weeks.

A Note on Calorie-Restricted Diets

We'd like to add a few words about calorie restriction and weight. One of the early signs of Alzheimer's disease is unexplained weight loss. One theory suggests that weight loss is due to the accumulation inside the brain of a peptide called amyloid-beta. This causes a disruption in the body's mechanism to regulate its weight, leading to accelerated weight loss years before an Alzheimer's diagnosis is made. Furthermore, many studies have found that the lower your caloric consumption throughout life, the lower your risk for developing Alzheimer's disease. The biology behind this is unclear, and more research is needed. This may be one more piece to the dietary puzzle in the prevention of Alzheimer's disease. For this reason, the calories in the following meal plans may seem a little low. For additional calories, adjust serving sizes or add vegetables, nuts, or high-protein foods. Also consider adding the suggested snacks to your daily intake.

Week 1

DAY 1

Breakfast

- 1 veggie omelet made with 2 eggs and 1 cup steamed or sautéed vegetables (such as red bell pepper, mushrooms, onion, kale, parsley, and thyme)
- ½ cup sweet potato hash browns
- ½ whole-grain English muffin
- ½ cup grapes (red or purple)
- Coffee

OPTIONAL ADDITIONS: top the omelet with ½ ounce cheese and/or ¼ cup salsa

Lunch

- 1½ cups Thai coconut curry soup with vegetables, garbanzo beans, and brown rice
- 1 plum, sliced
- Hot green tea with lemon

OPTIONAL ADDITIONS: 2 to 3 ounces steamed or baked tofu, shrimp, fish, or chicken in the curry; Thai chile pepper

Dinner

- Salad made with 4 ounces wild salmon with walnut pesto served on 2 cups fresh spinach dressed with 2 tablespoons vinaigrette made with fresh cilantro and apple cider vinegar
- 1 tomato, sliced
- 1 whole-grain roll with apricot compote

- 1 (6-ounce) glass of red wine

OPTIONAL ADDITIONS: 1 tablespoon Gorgonzola cheese and 1 sliced pear or apple on the salad

Dessert

- 1 (2-inch by 2-inch) square of spice cake
  (with added cardamom and chopped hazelnuts)

Snack (choose one)

- ½ cup raspberries
- 1 cup jicama and carrot sticks
- ¾ cup plain Greek yogurt
- ¼ cup almonds

DAY 2

Breakfast

- 2 tablespoons peanut or nut butter on 1 slice
  100 percent whole-grain (spelt) toast
- 1 cup kefir smoothie with cacao
- 1 fried plantain (use in the smoothie or sliced
  on top of the nut butter toast)
- Coffee

Lunch

- Salad made with 1 cup roasted beet cubes,
  2 cups arugula or beet greens, ½ cup berries, ½ cup
  grapefruit segments, and ⅛ cup pistachios, dressed with
  2 tablespoons vinaigrette (such as pomegranate)
- 1 small pumpkin muffin made with wheat germ
- Iced green tea or iced hibiscus tea

OPTIONAL ADDITIONS: 4 ounces tofu, ½ cup beans, and/or 1 tablespoon blue cheese crumbles on the salad

Dinner

- Stuffed red bell pepper filled with 1 cup mixed amaranth, white beans, thyme, and rosemary and topped with ½ cup marinara sauce
- 1 cup sautéed chard or other greens with garlic, chile peppers, and balsamic vinegar

OPTIONAL ADDITION: 1 tablespoon Pecorino Romano cheese on the stuffed pepper

Snack (choose one)

- 1 small orange
- 1 cup cucumber dressed with apple cider vinegar
- 1 cup steamed edamame (in shell)
- 1 hardboiled egg

DAY 3

Breakfast

- 1 cup hot millet porridge with cinnamon and nutmeg
- ¾ cup plain Greek yogurt
- ½ cup blueberries and raspberries
- 2 tablespoons pecans
- Coffee

Lunch

- 2 cups brown rice salad bowl with mung beans, avocado, cucumber, and tomatoes
- ½ cup pineapple chunks
- Hot cinnamon tea

Dinner

- 3 to 4 ounces Chilean sea bass, steamed or baked with fresh ginger and citrus
- 1 (4-inch-by-4-inch) piece baked winter squash with freshly ground black pepper
- 2 cups leafy green salad with added vegetables and ⅛ cup dressing of choice

Dessert

- ½ cup cherry crisp with topping of oats, nuts, and cacao

Snack (choose one)

- ½ cup peaches
- ¼ cup guacamole on tomato slices
- 2 tablespoons sunflower seeds
- 1 string cheese

DAY 4

Breakfast

- Mexican egg scramble made with 2 eggs and ½ cup mixed pinto beans, and 1 cup of onion, red bell pepper, zucchini, and spinach
- ¼ cup salsa
- 1 slice whole-grain toast
- ½ cup strawberry-cranberry compote
- Coffee

OPTIONAL ADDITIONS: ½ ounce shredded cheese and/or 1 tablespoon sour cream for the egg scramble

Lunch

- ½ cup tofu sautéed with soy sauce, sesame oil, and ginger; ½ cup rice noodles; cilantro; and chopped water chestnuts, wrapped in 3 napa cabbage leaves
- 1 whole grapefruit (2 fruit servings)
- Hot green tea with ginger

OPTIONAL ADDITIONS: Garlic chili sauce on the napa wraps; substitute ground chicken for the tofu

Dinner

- 1 (3- to 4-ounce) grilled bison or black bean burger with 1 tablespoon fresh horseradish sour cream
- ¼ cup shiitake mushrooms sautéed with fresh garlic
- 1 cup cooked farro with chopped vegetables
- 1 cup steamed collard greens with apple cider vinegar and black pepper
- 1 (12-ounce) glass craft beer brown ale

Snack (choose one)

- 1 small peach
- 1 cup snap peas
- ¼ cup cashews
- ½ cup cottage cheese with cumin and salsa

DAY 5

Breakfast

- 2 small buckwheat pancakes topped with chopped mango, ¾ cup plain Greek yogurt, and 2 tablespoons walnuts
- 4 ounces pomegranate juice
- 1 cup dark chocolate mocha

Lunch

- 1½ cups potato (sweet or regular) and leek soup topped with chopped sage
- ½ Reuben sandwich on whole-grain bread (with ½ cup sauerkraut and 2 ounces turkey or tofu)
- ½ cup red grapes and honeydew melon with lime zest
- Hot mint green tea

Dinner

- Fish taco made with 1 whole-grain or corn tortilla; 3 ounces whitefish baked with cumin and red bell pepper; 1 cup red cabbage, carrot, cilantro, and poblano slaw; and ½ cup black or pinto beans
- ¼ cup salsa
- 1 orange

OPTIONAL MODIFICATION: Transform this to a large salad by omitting the tortilla and adding 1 tablespoon sour cream, ½ ounce shredded cheese, sliced jalapeño, and more greens if you would like

Snack (choose one)

- Apple slices sprinkled with nutmeg
- 1 cup sliced bell pepper trio (red, orange, yellow)
- ½ cup kale chips
- 2 ounces sardines

DAY 6

Breakfast

- 2 poached eggs
- 1 cup red flannel hash made with beets, onions, and potatoes
- ½ whole-grain English muffin
- ½ cup plain nonfat yogurt with ½ cup fruit
- Coffee

Lunch

- ½ avocado filled with artichoke hearts, cucumber, and tomato, or tuna salad with red grapes
- 1 cup tomato-basil soup with freshly grated horseradish
- 6 whole-grain or flaxseed crackers
- ½ cup apricots
- Hot green tea with turmeric

Dinner

- 2 cups Moroccan-style lentil stew made with bulgur, carrots, cauliflower, turmeric, cinnamon, and cumin
- 1 small buckwheat roll
- 2 cups arugula and tomato salad with 2 tablespoons vinaigrette
- 1 (6-ounce) glass red wine

Dessert

- ½ cup mango cobbler sprinkled with chia seeds

Snack (choose one)

- 1 pear sprinkled with cardamom
- Steamed asparagus sticks with freshly squeezed lemon juice
- 2 tablespoons pumpkin seeds
- ½ cup frozen Greek yogurt

DAY 7

Breakfast

○ Yogurt parfait made with 1 cup plain Greek yogurt, ½ cup fresh fruit, ½ cup homemade granola made with toasted millet or bulgur, 1 tablespoon flaxseeds, and 1 tablespoon almonds

○ Coffee

OPTIONAL ADDITIONS: Top the parfait with 1 teaspoon strawberry preserves or honey

Lunch

○ 1 (6-inch) whole-grain flatbread with balsamic-glazed Brussels sprouts, leeks, squash, and Pecorino cheese

○ 2 cups cucumber and watercress salad with ½ cup garbanzo beans, 1 tablespoon pumpkin seeds, and 2 tablespoons vinaigrette

○ 1 orange

○ Iced green tea

OPTIONAL ADDITION: ½ ounce blue cheese crumbles on salad

Dinner

○ 3 to 4 ounces butterfish with 2 tablespoons chimichurri sauce

○ ½ cup mashed potatoes, sweet or regular

○ 1 cup steamed red cabbage with apple cider vinegar

○ 1 plum, sliced

Snack (choose one)

○ ½ cup melon cubes with fresh mint

○ 1 cup zucchini sticks

○ ¼ cup hazelnuts

○ ¼ cup white bean spread

Week 2

DAY 1

Breakfast

- Breakfast burrito made with 1 (6-inch) whole-grain tortilla, scrambled eggs, turmeric and cumin, ½ cup beans (such as black or pinto), and 1 chopped tomato
- 1 cup latte with cinnamon

OPTIONAL ADDITIONS: ½ ounce shredded cheese and/or ¼ cup mango salsa on burrito

Lunch

- 2 cups kale and basil salad topped with ¼ cup dried cranberries or raisins, ½ cup toasted millet or bulgur, 2 tablespoons chopped nuts, and 2 tablespoons dressing of choice
- 1 small peach
- Lavender green tea

OPTIONAL ADDITIONS: 2 ounces sardines and 1 tablespoon feta cheese on the salad

Dinner

- Spaghetti with meat(less)balls, made with 1 cup whole-grain pasta; ½ cup marinara sauce with rosemary, thyme, basil, garlic; and 4 ounces ground turkey meatballs or meatless meatballs
- 1 cup sautéed vegetables of choice (such as garlic, green beans, and carrots)
- 2 cups salad made with 1½ cups sliced fennel and ½ cup grapefruit segments with 2 tablespoons vinaigrette
- 1 (6-ounce) glass red wine

OPTIONAL ADDITION: 1 tablespoon Parmesan cheese on the pasta

Snack (choose one)

- 1 nectarine
- 1 cup pickled beets
- 1 tablespoon chia seeds on ½ cup plain Greek or regular yogurt
- ½ cup curry-spiced roasted garbanzo beans

DAY 2

Breakfast

- 2 small pumpkin pancakes with pumpkin seeds
- ½ cup cinnamon applesauce
- 1 (3- to 4-ounce) black bean patty
- Coffee

Lunch

- 1½ cups vegetable fried rice (brown) with tofu
- 1½ cups sautéed kale with ginger and garlic
- 1 small pear sprinkled with nutmeg
- Hot citrus green tea

Dinner

- 3 to 4 ounces blackened sablefish or wild salmon (rub made with garlic, chile pepper, black pepper, thyme, and cumin)
- 1 cup black-eyed peas and dandelion greens with 1 ounce feta cheese
- 1 cup steamed broccoli and okra with lemon zest
- ½ cup honeydew melon
- 1 (6-ounce) glass red wine or 1 (12-ounce) glass IPA craft beer

Dessert

- 1 lavender and lemon cookie

Snack (choose one)

o ½ cup cantaloupe cubes

o ½ cup roasted kohlrabi sprinkled with turmeric

o ¼ cup mixed nuts

o ¾ cup mango-berry smoothie

DAY 3

Breakfast

o 1 (3-by-3-inch) egg bake made with 2 eggs and
   1 cup sautéed vegetables of choice

o ½ cup blueberries with 1 tablespoon chopped pistachios

o 1 slice whole-grain toast

o 4 ounces fresh mango juice

o Coffee

OPTIONAL ADDITIONS: ½ ounce shredded cheese and ¼ cup salsa
on the egg bake

Lunch

o Grilled sandwich made with 2 slices whole-grain bread,
   ¼ cup hummus with wasabi, 1 portabello mushroom,
   1 thick slice eggplant, tomato, avocado, and spinach

o ½ cup cherries with cacao shavings and cinnamon

o Chamomile tea

Dinner

o 1 medium baked (regular or sweet) potato stuffed with 1 cup chili
   with beans (prepared with stout beer), 1 cup freshly chopped
   veggies (such as tomatoes, scallions, jicama), and ¼ cup salsa

o Leafy green salad with 2 tablespoons dressing of choice

OPTIONAL ADDITIONS: 2 tablespoons guacamole, ½ ounce shredded
cheese, and/or 1 tablespoon sour cream on the potato

Snack (choose one)

○ ½ banana

○ ½ cup roasted Brussels sprouts with rosemary

○ ¼ cup peanuts

○ ½ cup Greek yogurt

DAY 4

Breakfast

○ 1 cup cooked oatmeal topped with chia seeds, black currants, walnuts, and shredded coconut

○ 8 ounces kefir

○ ½ cup berries of choice with fresh mint

○ Coffee

Lunch

○ 1½ cups split pea soup with potatoes, kohlrabi, carrots, and leeks

○ 1 roll, 100 percent whole grain

○ 1 cup kale chips seasoned with turmeric and black pepper

○ ½ cup fruit salad

○ Iced green tea with 1 orange slice

Dinner

○ Open-faced sandwich made with 4 ounces trout baked (with chopped parsley and lime), and 1 slice whole-grain (spelt) bread

○ Salad made with 2 cups spinach, ½ cup blueberries, 2 tablespoons chopped almonds, and 2 tablespoons apple cider vinaigrette

OPTIONAL ADDITION: ½ ounce Gorgonzola cheese on the salad

Snack (choose one)

- 1 small orange
- 1 cup carrot and celery sticks
- ¼ cup pecans
- ¼ cup roasted red pepper hummus

DAY 5

Breakfast

- 1 (3-by-3-inch) egg and artichoke frittata with rosemary and basil
- 1 slice zucchini walnut bread with chia seeds or flaxseeds
- ½ cup sliced apricots or apricot compote
- Coffee

OPTIONAL ADDITION: ½ ounce cream cheese on the walnut bread

Lunch

- Bean and vegetable stew made with 1½ cups mixed vegetables and ½ cup beans
- 5 or 6 small whole-grain or flaxseed crackers
- 1 cup cucumber and asparagus salad
- Green tea with licorice root

OPTIONAL ADDITION: 2 to 3 ounces beef or tofu in the stew

Dinner

- ½ (5- to 6-inch) baked pumpkin stuffed with 1 cup barley and mixed mushrooms, with mint and curry
- 2 cups cabbage and kale salad with garlic, lemon, and extra-virgin olive oil
- 1 (12-ounce) glass craft wheat beer

Dessert

- ○ 4 dark chocolate–dipped strawberries

Snack (choose one)

- ○ 1 small bunch grapes (red or purple)
- ○ ½ cup cucumber slices, tomatoes, and olives
- ○ ¼ cup toasted almonds with turmeric
- ○ ½ cup cottage cheese or yogurt on celery

DAY 6

Breakfast

- ○ 1 cup whole-grain and flaxseed cold cereal with milk
- ○ ½ banana with 2 tablespoons peanut or nut butter
- ○ ¾ cup plain Greek yogurt with ½ cup raspberries
- ○ Coffee

Lunch Out

- ○ 1 (8-piece) Unagi sushi roll (eel, cucumber, avocado, brown rice) with wasabi, soy sauce, and pickled ginger
- ○ 1 cup seaweed salad
- ○ 1 cup miso soup
- ○ 1 cup edamame (in shell) sprinkled with garlic salt and red pepper flakes
- ○ Hot green jasmine tea

Dinner

- 1 cup spinach ravioli with roasted garlic and sun-dried tomatoes
- 1 (4-by-4-inch) piece baked Hubbard squash with sage
- Salad made with 2 cups arugula with chopped figs, ½ ounce mozzarella, and ½ cup cherry tomatoes, dressed with 2 tablespoons basic vinaigrette
- ½ cup melon
- 1 (6-ounce) glass red wine

Snack (choose one)

- ½ cup pineapple chunks with chili powder
- ½ cup three-bean salad
- ¼ cup curry-roasted cashews
- 2 ounces chilled shrimp with horseradish cocktail sauce

DAY 7

Breakfast

- 1 cup egg, farro, and vegetable hash
- ½ cup corn and black bean salsa
- 1 slice whole-grain toast
- ½ cup pomegranate juice
- Coffee

OPTIONAL ADDITIONS: ½ ounce shredded cheese and/or 1 tablespoon sour cream on the hash

Lunch

- Two pieces of pizza made with 1 (12-inch) whole-grain crust, tomatoes, fresh garlic, basil, thyme, parsley, shiitake and other mushrooms, Kalamata and green olives, red bell pepper, and low-fat mozzarella cheese
- 1 cup wilted spinach salad dressed with balsamic or apple cider vinegar
- Iced ginger green tea

Dinner

- 1 (1-inch-thick) grilled cauliflower steak with Romesco sauce (extra-virgin olive oil, roasted red bell pepper, garlic, and almonds)
- 1 cup white beans with chard
- 1 small baked potato or yam with fresh rosemary, thyme, and basil
- ½ cup fresh fruit

Dessert

- ½ cup blackberries on ½ cup lemon sorbet or sherbet

Snack (choose one)

- ½ cup grapefruit and orange segments
- 1 steamed artichoke with freshly squeezed lime juice
- 2 tablespoons roasted pumpkin seeds with freshly ground black pepper
- 1 deviled egg with apple cider vinegar

Brain-Healthy Food Combinations

Meal planning and food pairing do not have to be rocket science, but there is a little culinary wizardry involved. One of the secrets in successfully combining foods is to think in terms of opposites. When the main dish is complicated, keep the vegetable simple. If most of the meal is dark and rich (as in roasted vegetables), balance this out with a light salad. If it's light, like a fresh Caesar salad, add a little weight with a slice of whole-grain bread. Think seasonal. Shop for

Spices	Vegetable	Fruit	Protein	
Basil	Artichoke, chile pepper, eggplant, okra, red bell pepper, zucchini	Apricot, berries, plum	All protein sources	
Black Pepper	All vegetables	Citrus	Eggs, fish, nuts, seeds, tofu	
Cacao		Apricot, berries, cherries, citrus, grapes (red or purple), mango, plantain	Any protein when used with other Mexican spices, yogurt	
Cardamom	Mushrooms, pumpkin, sweet potato, winter squash	Mango	Garbanzo beans, legumes, nuts, yogurt	
Chamomile	Leafy greens	Citrus, melon		
Cinnamon	Carrot, pumpkin, squash, sweet potato, yam	Apricot	Black-eyed peas, lentils, nuts, tofu	

produce in season and build your meals around the freshest of ingredients. For a taste sensation, use this chart to pair brain foods with spices; the more you try, the better you will become at combining flavors and nutrients.

Foods that nourish and protect your brain from Alzheimer's disease are colorful, flavorful, and easy to combine with your own family favorites. Enjoy them!

	Grain	Craft Beer	Wine	Tea
	All grains	Pilsner, lager	Soave, gavi, pinot grigio	Green tea
	All grains	Bock	Cabernet sauvignon, syrah, petite syrah, port	
	Oats	Lager	Sweet red wines	All teas, coffee
	Brown rice, millet, oats	Wheat beers	Viognier, zinfandel	Coffee
			Zinfandel, Amarone	All teas
	Brown rice, all grains		All bold red wines	All teas, coffee

Spices	Vegetable	Fruit	Protein	
Cilantro	Avocado, chile pepper, leek, red bell pepper	Mango, plantain	All beans, garbanzo beans, lentils, mung beans	
Cumin	Avocado, Brussels sprouts, carrot, cabbage, cucumber, kohlrabi, tomato	Citrus, mango	Fish, black-eyed peas, garbanzo beans, lentils, mung beans	
Ginger	Broccoli, Brussels sprouts, carrot, kohlrabi, pumpkin	Citrus, mango	Fish, black-eyed peas, garbanzo beans, lentils, mung beans	
Horseradish	Leafy greens, root vegetables, tomato		Eggs, fish	
Lavender	Leafy greens, potato	Berries, citrus	Combined with citrus on fish	
Licorice	Leafy greens, jicama	Cherries	Mung beans, beans	
Mint	Beans, cucumber, carrot, eggplant, zucchini	Apricot, berries, citrus, cherries, plum	Fish, garbanzo beans, lentils, yogurt	
Nutmeg	Asparagus, broccoli, cabbage, carrot, cauliflower, mushrooms, sweet potato, spinach	Mango, pomegranate	Fish, tofu	
Parsley	Cucumber, carrot, eggplant, zucchini, root vegetables, tomato	Mango, plantain, grapefruit	Fish, lentils	
Rosemary	Asparagus, beet, mushrooms, root vegetables, tomato	Citrus	All protein sources	

	Grain	Craft Beer	Wine	Tea
	All grains	Pilsner, IPA		
	All grains	Pilsner, IPA, saison	Sparkling rosé, Bordeaux	
		Wheat beers	Riesling, sauternes	All teas
	Brown rice, spelt	Brown ale	Riesling	
	Amaranth, brown rice		Monastrell, rosé, gewürztraminer	All teas
			Barbera, syrah	All teas
	All grains	Saison	Riesling, merlot, moscato	Green tea
	Millet, oats	Wheat beers	All bold red wines	All teas
	All grains	Wheat beers, saison		Green tea
	All grains	Wheat beers	Shiraz, zinfandel	Green tea

Spices	Vegetable	Fruit	Protein	
Sage	Beet, carrot, kohlrabi, leek, mushrooms, potato, pumpkin, sweet potato, winter squash, yam, zucchini	Citrus, plum	Fish, nuts	
Thyme	Artichoke, beet, broccoli, cauliflower, mushrooms, tomato, zucchini	Cherries, citrus, grapes (red and purple)	All protein sources	
Turmeric	Beet, Brussels sprouts, carrot, cauliflower, mushrooms, potato, sweet potato, yam	Berries, citrus	Black-eyed peas, lentils, nuts	
Wasabi	Cucumber, leafy greens, potato, root vegetables		Fish, nuts	

	Grain	Craft Beer	Wine	Tea
	All grains	Saison	Riesling	Green tea
	Brown rice, millet, oats	Saison	Pinot noir, zweigelt	Green tea
	All grains	IPA	Chardonnay, Sémillon	All teas
	Brown rice	Pilsner, wheat beers	Chenin blanc	

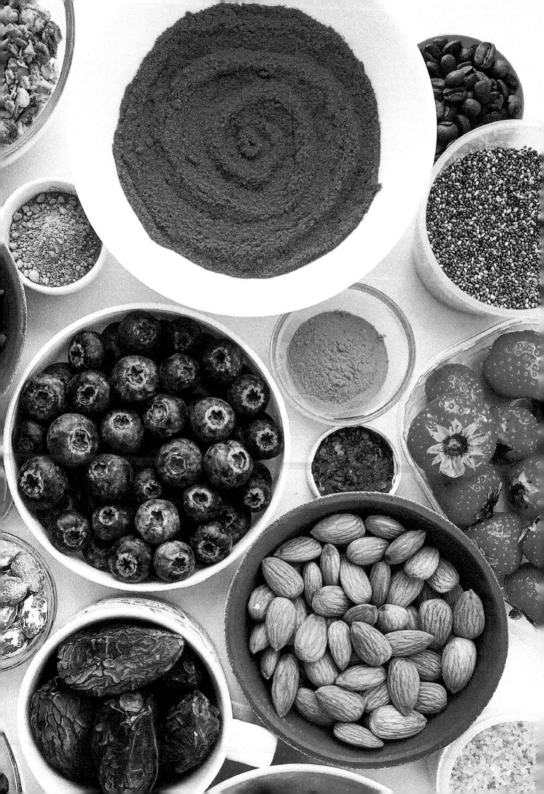

Appendix A
Tips for a Healthy Lifestyle

The diet we eat is considered a modifiable risk factor for the development of Alzheimer's disease. Modifiable risks are the lifestyle hazards we actually have control over, such as the decision to eat brain-healthy foods or follow a meat-sweet diet. While dietary changes are key, lifestyle is also very important for the maintenance of a healthy mind. Sleep, stress management, and exercise are also modifiable risk factors for the prevention of this debilitating disease. Consider making changes in these areas to promote your overall healthy lifestyle.

Good Sleep

If you toss and turn all night, go to bed late and get up early, or find yourself so tired during the day that you are irritable and unproductive, you may not be getting the kind of sleep your brain needs. We spend a third of our lives asleep (or we should), yet we don't give sleep the credit it deserves.

Over the years, a number of studies have linked sleep patterns to cognition and Alzheimer's disease. Individuals with known sleep disorders have a higher likelihood of developing dementia, and those with dementia have more sleep disturbances. Research from Johns Hopkins University showed an increase in amyloid protein and plaques (damaging buildup found in Alzheimer's patients leading to decreased cognition and brain shrinkage) in the brains of patients reporting the most sleep disturbances. Studies are ongoing to help determine if poor sleep causes amyloid deposition or if amyloid plaques disrupt sleep. In some patients with sleep issues, chamomile tea or melatonin can be helpful supplements.

Sleep tips:

- Sleep 7 to 8 hours a night.
- Limit daytime naps to 30 minutes.
- Exercise daily to promote good-quality sleep—but exercising right before bedtime might disrupt sleep, so plan to get your steps in early.
- Steer clear of foods known to disrupt sleep: Rich foods, fatty foods, spicy foods, citrus, and carbonated beverages may disrupt a good night's sleep.
- Avoid caffeinated beverages in the evenings. If you drink alcohol, do so in moderation for the best sleep outcome.
- Certain foods, especially those high in magnesium, calcium, potassium, and vitamin B_6, may help promote good sleep. Many foods in this guidebook are chock-full of these nutrients. Some examples of foods you can eat at the evening meal or have as a light bedtime snack on occasion include tart cherries, plantains or bananas, fish, jasmine brown rice, and yogurt (or warm milk like your grandmother used). Also, chamomile tea has been used for centuries to induce sleep.
- Expose yourself to a good dose of natural light during the day to maintain a healthy sleep-wake cycle.
- Establish relaxing bedtime routines. This may include taking a hot bath or reading.

- Minimize noise (unless it's white noise from a humidifier or fan), bright lights, and electronic screens. It is a good idea to put your phone and other digital devices out of sight and out of reach.
- A comfortable bed and pillow also make a world of difference in promoting great sleep.

Stress Management

Did you know that stress, worry, and anxiety may disrupt normal brain function and increase your risk for Alzheimer's disease? While we don't want this news to stress you out, it might be time to take control of your life and reduce the stress.

Cortisol is a life-sustaining hormone produced by the adrenal glands. It is released in times of stress and is a positive mechanism that helps us cope. However, when stress is long-lasting or chronic, the ongoing production of cortisol affects the memory and learning center in the hippocampus region of the brain. The hippocampus shrinks when cortisol levels stay high, and as a result this important part of the brain cannot do its job. The long-term result can be devastating—memory loss and perhaps Alzheimer's dementia.

Many ways exist to limit life's stressors. Avoiding stressful situations is ideal, and it is important to try to do this whenever possible. Meditation, yoga, breathing sequences, exercise, prayer, and daily affirmations are some ways to deal with stress. Eating a diet built around brain-healthy foods and getting great sleep are crucial as well. Remember that stress reduction does not happen overnight; if you incorporate things like meditation into your daily routine, the positive effects are cumulative and will result in a decreased risk of Alzheimer's disease and a more serene you.

Stretching and Exercise

According to the Alzheimer's Research and Prevention Foundation, regular physical activity can reduce your risk of developing Alzheimer's disease by 50 percent. Exercise causes increased blood flow to the brain, providing nourishment, slowing cognitive decline, and improving memory. It also helps reduce stress and improves sleep.

Current recommendations for exercise to promote a healthy heart and brain include incorporating 150 minutes of movement per week. Another approach is to do 30 minutes per day, which can be broken up into three 10-minute sessions. Your physical activity should be moderately strenuous and should raise your heart rate. Additionally, stretching is important for balance and flexibility. Activity ideas include swimming, tai chi, yoga, team sports, and walking.

Movement tips:

- Always warm up and cool down—start each exercise routine slowly to avoid injury.
- Replace a coffee break with a brisk 10-minute walk.
- Include weight-bearing exercises at least three times per week to decrease the risk of falls.
- Turn sit time into fit time—incorporate stretches and exercise you can do at your desk or while sitting on the couch into your daily routine.
- Exercise with a friend or listen to something mind stimulating while you work out.

Fasting at Night

Emerging research from UCLA supports the benefits of fasting for a minimum of 12 hours between dinner and breakfast. Fasting can decrease inflammation, decrease oxidative stress, and assist the body in using ketones for energy. As noted previously, the use of ketones for energy may be a key link to reducing cognitive decline. Eat your dinner meal early and reduce evening snacking to start a nighttime fasting routine.

Appendix B
Glossary

Alzheimer's disease: The most common form of neurodegenerative disorder affecting memory, thinking, and behavior. It is characterized by the gradual loss of neurons and synapses in the brain and eventually leads to death.

anti-inflammatory: Reducing or counteracting inflammation.

antioxidants: Various substances that inhibit cell oxidation or reactions promoted by oxidizing agents in a living organism.

brain health: The brain's ability to perform all the mental processes collectively known as cognition, including learning ability, intuition, judgment, language, and memory.

brain response time: Skill and knowledge to acquire factual information, often in a time period that can be measured. Also known as cognitive response.

carotenoids: The various yellow, orange, red, and green pigments found in many fruits and vegetables. The two main types are carotenes and xanthophylls. Carotenes are typically yellow and orange, and beta-carotene is a well-known carotene in foods such as carrots, spinach, and apricots.

cell regeneration: The process of renewal, restoration, and growth that makes cells resilient to natural fluctuations or events that cause disturbance or damage.

cognitive function: An intellectual process by which one becomes aware of, perceives, or comprehends ideas. It involves all aspects of perception, thinking, reasoning, and remembering.

flavonoids: A group of plant metabolites thought to provide health benefits through cell signaling pathways and antioxidant effects. Examples are isoflavonoids, anthoxanthins, and anthocyanins.

free radicals: These are molecules with unpaired electrons. They rob other cells of electrons, causing damage and contributing toward many diseases.

gray matter: Nerve tissue, especially of the brain and spinal cord, that contains fibers and nerve cell bodies and is dark reddish-gray.

homocysteine: An amino acid produced by the body if elevated is a marker measured in the blood for cardiovascular disease and increased risk of Alzheimer's disease.

ketosis: A metabolic process that occurs when the body does not have enough glucose for energy. This causes stored fat to be broken down for energy, resulting in a buildup of acids, called ketones, within the body.

memory: The ability of the mind to store and remember information.

mental clarity: A state of emotional and psychological well-being in which an individual is able to use his or her cognitive and emotional capabilities, function in society, and meet the ordinary demands of everyday life.

nerve function: The ability of a bundle of nerves to use electrical and chemical signals to transmit sensory and motor information from one body part to another.

omega-3 fatty acids: A class of essential fatty acids needed in the human body. The body cannot produce them on its own, so they must be obtained from the diet. There are three main types of omega-3 fatty acids: ALA, DHA, and EPA.

oxidation: The process of eroding electrons. For example, when metal rusts, oxygen is stealing electrons from iron. Oxygen levels are reduced while iron in cells is oxidized.

phytochemicals: Non-nutritive plant chemicals that have protective or disease-preventive properties and are often responsible for the plant's color. Also called phytonutrients.

polyphenols: Phytochemicals that act as antioxidants.

reasoning: The ability of the mind to think and understand things in a logical way.

resveratrol: A polyphenol compound with antioxidant properties found in certain plants and in red wine.

sleep enhancement: Something that helps, augments, or improves the ability to sleep.

tau protein: A protein abundant in the neurons of the central nervous system. The abnormal function of tau and tangles leads to neurodegenerative disorders such as Alzheimer's disease.

trans fatty acids: An unsaturated fatty acid found in margarines, manufactured cooking oils, and processed foods. Consumption is thought to increase blood lipids and the risk of cardiovascular disease.

Appendix C
Resources

Academy of Nutrition and Dietetics
https://www.eatright.org

Alzheimer's Association
http://www.alz.org

Alzheimer's Foundation of America
http://www.alzfdn.org

Alzheimer's Research Worldwide
http://www.alz.org/research/overview.asp

Alzheimer's Society—UK
https://www.alzheimers.org.uk

Ask For Evidence—Sense About Science
http://askforevidence.org/help/alzheimers-dementia-knowledge-bank

Banner Alzheimer's Institute
http://banneralz.org

Bright Focus Foundation
http://www.brightfocus.org/alzheimers/article
/what-your-risk-heredity-and-late-onset-alzheimers-disease

Dietitians of Canada—PEN Nutrition
http://www.pennutrition.com/index.aspx

Eating Well
http://www.eatingwell.com

Fisher Center for Alzheimer's Research
https://www.alzinfo.org

Harvard School of Public Health
https://www.hsph.harvard.edu

Inflammation Research Foundation
http://www.inflammationresearchfoundation.org

Mayo Clinic—Alzheimer's Disease Research Center
http://www.mayo.edu/research/centers-programs
/alzheimers-disease-research-center

Medline Plus
https://medlineplus.gov

National Institute of Neurological Disorders and Stroke
https://www.ninds.nih.gov

National Institute on Aging
https://www.nia.nih.gov/alzheimers

Neurobiology of Aging
http://www.neurobiologyofaging.org

Neurology Today
http://journals.lww.com/neurotodayonline/

Old Ways—Mediterranean Diet
http://www.oldwayspt.org

Oregon Health and Science University—Aging and Alzheimer's
Disease Center
http://www.ohsu.edu/xd/research/centers-institutes/neurology
/alzheimers/

Pub Med
https://www.ncbi.nlm.nih.gov/pubmed/

Today's Dietitian
http://www.todaysdietitian.com

Tuft's University Health and Nutrition Newsletter
http://www.nutritionletter.tufts.edu

UCLA Brain Research Institute
http://www.bri.ucla.edu

USDA Food Composition Database
https://ndb.nal.usda.gov/ndb/

The World's Healthiest Foods
http://www.whfoods.com

Bibliography

11 proven health benefits of ginger. (2016, August 18). Retrieved January 11, 2017, from https://authoritynutrition.com/11-proven-benefits -of-ginger/.

2016 Alzheimer's disease facts and figures fact sheet. (2016). Retrieved January 10, 2017, from www.alz.org/documents_custom /2016-facts-and-figures.pdf.

About Alzheimer's disease: Alzheimer's basics. (n.d.). Retrieved January 10, 2017, from www.nia.nih.gov/alzheimers/topics/alzheimers-basics.

Aggarwal, B. B. (2010). Targeting inflammation-induced obesity and metabolic diseases by curcumin and other nutraceuticals. *Annual Revue of Nutrition, 30,* 173–199.

Aisen, P. S., Schneider, L. S., Sano, M., Diaz-Arrastia, R., van Dyck, C. H., Weiner, M. F. . . . Thal, L. J. (2008). High-dose B vitamin supplementation and cognitive decline in Alzheimer disease: a randomized controlled trial. *Journal of the American Medical Association, 300,* 1774–1783.

Almonds. (n.d.). Retrieved January 11, 2017, from www.whfoods.com /genpage.php?tname=foodspice&dbid=20.

Alzheimer's Brain Tangles—Alzheimer's Association. (n.d.). Retrieved January 10, 2017, from www.alz.org/braintour/tangles.asp.

Alzheimer's Society (n.d.). A novel approach to protecting nerve cells in Alzheimer's disease. Retrieved January 11, 2017, from www.alzheimers .org.uk/site/scripts/documents_info.php?documentID=1131.

American Chemical Society. (2016, March 14). Blueberries, the well-known "super fruit," could help fight Alzheimer's. Retrieved January 11, 2017, from www.sciencedaily.com/releases/2016/03/160314084821.htm.

Andrea, T., Angeloni, C., Malaguti, M., Fabiana, M., Hrelia, S., & Patrizia, H. (2014). Sulforaphane as a potential protective phytochemical against neurodegenerative diseases. *Front Aging Neuroscience, 6*, 282.

Anekonda, T. S. (2006). Resveratrol—a boon for treating Alzheimer's disease? *Brain Research Reviews, 52,* 316–326.

Anekonda, T. S., Reddy P. H. (2006). Neuronal protection by sirtuins in Alzheimer's disease. *Journal of Neurochemistry, 96,* 305–313.

Anthocyanins. (2014, March). www.todaysdietitian.com /newarchives/030314p20.shtml.

Apricots. (n.d.). Retrieved January 11, 2017, from www.whfoods.com /genpage.php?tname=foodspice&dbid=3.

Avocados. (n.d.). Retrieved January 11, 2017, from www.whfoods.com /genpage.php?tname=foodspice&dbid=5.

Baum, L., Lam, C. W., Cheung, S. K., Kwok, T., Lui, V., Tsoh, J. . . . Mok, V. (2008). Six-month randomized, placebo-controlled, double-blind, pilot clinical trial of curcumin in patients with Alzheimer disease. *Journal of Clinical Psychopharmacology,* 28, 110–113.

Baur, J. A., Pearson, K. J., Price, N. L., Jamieson, H. A., Lerin, C., Kalra, A. . . . Sinclair, D. A. (2006). Resveratrol improves health and survival of mice on a high-calorie diet. *Nature, 444,* 337–342.

Beer lovers rejoice. (n.d.). Retrieved March 9, 2017, from www .nutritionsecrets.com/health-benefits-beer/.

Beet greens nutrition facts and health benefits. (n.d.). Retrieved January 11, 2017, from www.nutrition-and-you.com/beet-greens.html.

Bendlin, B. B., Carlsson, C. M., Gleason, C. E., Johnson, S. C., Sodhi, A., Gallagher, C. L. . . . Asthana, S. (2010). Midlife predictors of Alzheimer's disease. *Maturitas, 65,* 131–137.

Beydoun, M. A., Kaufman, J. S., Satia, J. A., Rosamond, W., Folsom, A. R. (2007). Plasma n-3 fatty acids and the risk of cognitive decline in older adults: the atherosclerosis risk in communities study. *American Journal of Clinical Nutrition, 85,* 1103–1111.

Bhagavan, H. N., Chopra, R. K. (2006). Coenzyme Q10: absorption, tissue uptake, metabolism and pharmacokinetics. *Free Radical Research, 40,* 445–453.

Bharadwaj, P. R., Bates, K. A., Porter, T., Teimouri, E., Perry, G., Steele, J. W. . . . Verdile, G. (2013). Latrepirdine: molecular mechanisms underlying potential therapeutic roles in Alzheimer's and other neurodegenerative diseases. *Translational Psychiatry, 3,* e332.

Blackwell, T., Yaffe, K., Ancoli-Israel, S., Redline, S., Ensrud, K. E., Stefanick, M. L. . . . Stone, K. L. (2011). Association of sleep characteristics and cognition in older community-dwelling men: the MrOS sleep study. *Sleep, 34,* 1347–1356.

Blueberries. (n.d.). Retrieved January 11, 2017, from www.whfoods.com /genpage.php?tname=foodspice&dbid=8.

Blumberg, J., Heaney, R. P., Huncharek, M., Scholl, T., Stampfer, M., Vieth, R. . . . Zeisel, S. H. (2010). Evidence-based criteria in the nutritional context. *Nutritional Review, 68,* 478–484.

Bourdel-Marchasson, I., Delmas-Beauviex, M. C., Peuchant, E., Richard-Harston, S., Decamps, A., Regnier, B. . . . Rainfray, M. (2001). Antioxidant defenses and oxidative stress markers in erythrocytes and plasma from normally nourished elderly Alzheimer patients. *Age and Ageing, 30*(3), 235–241.

Bowman G. L. (2012). Ascorbic acid, cognitive function, and Alzheimer's disease: a current review and future direction. *Biofactors, 38,* 114–122.

Bredesen, D. E. (2014). Reversal of cognitive decline: a novel therapeutic program. *Aging. 6*(9), 707-717.

Brewer, G. J. (2009). The risks of copper toxicity contributing to cognitive decline in the aging population and Alzheimer's disease. *Journal of the American College of Nutrition, 28,* 238–242.

Broccoli. (n.d.). Retrieved January 10, 2017, from www.whfoods.com
/genpage.php?tname=foodspice&dbid=9.

Brookmeyer, R., Johnson, E., Ziegler-Graham, K., Arrighi, H. M. (2007).
Forecasting the global burden of Alzheimer's disease. *Alzheimers &
Dementia, 3*, 186–191.

Cabbage nutrition facts and health benefits. (n.d.). Retrieved January 10,
2017, from www.nutrition-and-you.com/cabbage.html.

Can spinach reduce the risk of dementia? (2015, April 24). Retrieved
January 10, 2017, from www.alzheimers.net/4-29-15-spinach
-reduces-dementia-risk/.

Cardoso, B. R., Cominetti, C., Cozzolino, S. M. (2013). Importance
and management of micronutrient deficiencies in patients with
Alzheimer's disease. *Journal of Clinical Interventions in Aging, 8,*
531–542.

Certain foods may protect against Alzheimer's disease. (2010).
Retrieved January 10, 2017, from www.alzinfo.org/articles
/certain-foods-may-protect-against-alzheimers-disease-2.

Choi, D. Y., Lee, Y. J., Hong, J. T., Lee, H. J. (2012). Antioxidant properties
of natural polyphenols and their therapeutic potentials
for Alzheimer's disease. *Brain Research Bulletin, 87*(2–3), 144–153.

Coconut oil. (n.d.). Retrieved March 9, 2017, from https://www.alzheimers
.org.uk/info/20074/alternative_therapies/119/coconut_oil.

Coconut oil nutrition facts and health benefits. (n.d.). Retrieved
January 13, 2017, from www.nutrition-and-you.com/coconut-oil.html.

Cognitive function. (2017, January 3). Retrieved January 10, 2017,
from http://lpi.oregonstate.edu/mic/health-disease
/cognitive-function#memory.

Cooking with spices: lavender. (n.d.). Retrieved March 9, 2017, from
www.drweil.com/diet-nutrition/cooking-cookware/cooking-with
-spices-lavender/.

Cooper, J. K. (2014). Nutrition and the brain: what advice should we give? *Neurobiology of Aging, 35,* S79–S83.

Cordain, L., Eaton, S. B., Sebastian, A., Mann, N., Lindeberg, S., Watkins, B. A. . . . Brand-Miller, J. (2005). Origins and evolution of the Western diet: health implications for the 21st century. *American Journal of Clinical Nutrition, 81,* 341–354.

Corona, C., Masciopinto, F., Silvestri, E., Viscovo A.D., Lattanzio, R., Sorda, R. L. . . . Sensi, S. L. (2010). Dietary zinc supplementation of 3xTg-AD mice increases BDNF levels and prevents cognitive deficits as well as mitochondrial dysfunction. *Cell Death & Disease, 1,* e91.

Could cabbage and broccoli help in the fight against Alzheimer's? (n.d.). Retrieved January 10, 2017, from www.urmc.rochester.edu/research /blog/april-2014/could-cabbage-and-broccoli-help-in-the-fight -again.aspx.

Craft, S., Cholerton, B., Baker, L. D. (2013). Insulin and Alzheimer's disease: untangling the web. *Journal of Alzheimer's Disease, 33* (Supplement 1), S263–S275.

Crapper, D. R., Kishnan, S. S., Dalton, A. J. (1973). Brain aluminum distribution in Alzheimer's disease and experimental neurofibrillary degeneration. *Science, 180,* 511–513.

Cunnane, S., Nugent, S., Roy, M., Courchesne-Loyer, A., Croteau, E., Tremblay S. . . . Rapoport, S. I. (2011). Brain fuel metabolism, aging, and Alzheimer's disease. *Nutrition, 27,* 3–20.

Dangour, A. D., Whitehouse, P. J., Rafferty, K., Mitchell, S. A., Smith, L., Hawkesworth, S., Vellas B. (2010). B-vitamins and fatty acids in the prevention and treatment of Alzheimer's disease and dementia: a systematic review. *Journal of Alzheimer's Disease, 22,* 205–224.

Daviglus, M. L., Plassman, B. L., Pirzada, A., Bell, C. C., Bowen, P. E., Burke, J. R. . . . Williams, J. W. Jr. (2011). Risk factors and preventive interventions for Alzheimer disease: state of the science. *Archives of Neurology, 68,* 1185–1190.

Davinelli, S., Sapere, N., Zella, D., Bracale, R., Intrieri, M., Scapagnini, G. (2012). Pleiotropic protective effects of phytochemicals in Alzheimer's disease. *Oxidative Medicine and Cellular Longevity,* 386527.

de Jager, C. A., Oulhaj, A., Jacoby, R., Refsum, H., Smith, A. D. (2012). Cognitive and clinical outcomes of lowering homocysteine-lowering B-vitamin treatment in mild cognitive impairment: a randomized controlled trial. *International Journal of Geriatric Psychiatry, 27,* 592–600.

de la Monte, S. M., Tong, M. (2014). Brain metabolic dysfunction at the core of Alzheimer's disease. *Biochemical Pharmacology, 88,* 548–559.

DeDea, L. (2012). Can coconut oil replace caprylidene for Alzheimer disease? *Journal of the American Academy of Physician Assistants, 25,* 19.

DeFina, L. F., Willis, B. L., Radford, N. B., Gao, A., Leonard, D., Haskell, W. . . . Berry, J. D. (2013). The association between midlife cardiorespiratory fitness levels and later-life dementia. A cohort study. *Annals of Internal Medicine, 158,* 162–168.

DeKosky, S. T., Williamson, J. D., Fitzpatrick, A. L., Kronmal, R. A., Ives, D. G., Saxton, J. A. . . . Furberg, C. D. (2008). Ginkgo biloba for prevention of dementia: a randomized controlled trial. *Journal of the American Medical Association, 300,* 2253–2262.

Devore, E. E., Goldstein, F., van Rooij, F. J., Hofman, A., Stampfer, M. J., Witteman, J. C., Breteler, M. M. (2010) Dietary antioxidants and long-term risk of dementia. *Archives of Neurology, 67*(7), 819–825.

Diabetes and Alzheimer's linked. (2016). Retrieved January 10, 2017, from www.mayoclinic.org/diseases-conditions/alzheimers-disease /in-depth/diabetes-and-alzheimers/art-20046987.

Diet and Alzheimer's disease. (n.d.). Retrieved March 9, 2017, from www.pcrm.org/health/health-topics/diet-and-alzheimers-disease.

Diet and Alzheimer's disease: what the evidence shows. (2017). Retrieved January 10, 2017, from www.medscape.com/viewarticle/466037.

Diet and the brain. (n.d.). Retrieved March 9, 2017, from www.hbo.com /alzheimers/science-diet-and-the-brain.html.

Don't skip strawberries! (2016). Retrieved March 9, 2017, from wexnermedical.osu.edu/blog/dietitian-weighs-in-on-dirty-dozen -fruits-and-vegetables.

Douaud, G., Refsum, H., de Jager, C. A., Jacoby, R., Nichols, T. E., Smith, S. M., Smith, A. D. (2013). Preventing Alzheimer's disease-related gray matter atrophy by B-vitamin treatment. *Proceedings of the National Academy of Sciences, 110,* 9523–9528.

Dysken, M. W., Sano, M., Asthana, S., Vertrees, J. E., Pallaki, M., Llorente, M., Guarino, P. D. (2014). Effect of vitamin E and memantine on functional decline in Alzheimer disease: the TEAM-AD VA cooperative randomized trial. *Journal of the American Medical Association, 311,* 33–44.

Eat grapes as part of a healthy Alzheimer's Diet. (2016, June 4). Retrieved January 11, 2017, from http://theadplan.com/alzheimersdietblog /alzheimers-diet-2/eat-grapes-as-part-of-a-healthy-alzheimers-diet/.

Eating more whole grains linked with lower mortality rates. (2016). Retrieved March 9, 2017, from www.hsph.harvard.edu/news /press-releases/whole-grains-lower-mortality-rates/.

Erickson, K. I., Weinstein, A. M., Lopez, O. L. (2012). Physical activity, brain plasticity, and Alzheimer's disease. *Archives of Medical Research, 43,* 615–621.

Falkingham, M., Abdelhamid, A., Curtis, P., Fairweather-Tait, S., Dye, L., and Hooper, L. (2010). The effects of oral iron supplementation on cognition in older children and adults: a systematic review and meta-analysis. *Nutrition Journal, 9*(1, article 4)

Fang, L., Gou, S., Liu, X., Cao, F., Cheng, L. (2014). Design, synthesis and anti-Alzheimer properties of dimethylaminomethyl-substituted curcumin derivatives. *Bioorganic & Medicinal Chemistry Letters, 24,* 40–43.

Farro perlato (triticum dicoccum) (Emmer wheat?) nutrition facts & calories. (n.d.). Retrieved January 11, 2017, from http://nutritiondata.self.com/facts/custom/3236857/2.

Feart, C., Samieri, C., Barberger-Gateau, P. (2010). Mediterranean diet and cognitive function in older adults. *Current Opinion in Clinical Nutrition and Metabolic Care, 13,* 14–18.

Federation of American Societies for Experimental Biology. (2015, March 30). Eating green leafy vegetables keeps mental abilities sharp. Retrieved January 10, 2017, from www.sciencedaily.com /releases/2015/03/150330112227.htm.

Filipcik, P., Cente, M., Ferencik, M., Hulin, I., Novak, M. (2006). The role of oxidative stress in the pathogenesis of Alzheimer's disease. *Bratislavské Lekárske Listy, 107,* 384–394.

Fish, flaxseed may lower Alzheimer's risk. (n.d.). Retrieved January 12, 2017, from www.webmd.com/alzheimers/news/20120502 /fish-flaxseed-may-lower-alzheimers-risk#1.

Fish: friend or foe? (n.d.). Retrieved March 9, 2017, from www.hsph .harvard.edu/nutritionsource/fish/#1.

Fisher, N. D., Sorond, F. A., Hollenberg, N. K. (2006). Cocoa flavanols and brain perfusion. *Journal of Cardiovascular Pharmacology, 47,* (Supplement 2), S210.

Flavonoids, cognition, and dementia: actions, mechanisms, and potential therapeutic utility for Alzheimer disease. (n.d.). Retrieved January 11, 2017, from www.ncbi.nlm.nih.gov/pubmed/21982844.

Freund-Levi, Y., Eriksdotter-Jönhagen, M., Cederholm, T., Basun, H., Faxén-Irving, G., Garlind, A. ... Palmblad, J. (2006). Omega-3 fatty acid treatment in 174 patients with mild to moderate Alzheimer disease: OmegAD study: a randomized double-blind trial. *Archives of Neurology, 63,* 1402–1408.

Frisardi, V., Solfrizzi, V., Seripa, D., Capurso, C., Santamato, A., Sancarlo, D. . . . Panza, F. (2010). Metabolic-cognitive syndrome: a cross-talk between metabolic syndrome and Alzheimer's disease. *Ageing Research Reviews, 9,* 399–417.

Galasko, D. R., Peskind, E., Clark, C. M., Quinn, J. F., Ringman, J. M., Jicha, G. A. . . . Aisen, P. (2012). Antioxidants for Alzheimer disease: a randomized clinical trial with cerebrospinal fluid biomarker measures. *Archives of Neurology, 69*(7), 836–841.

Garbanzo beans (chickpeas). (n.d.). Retrieved January 11, 2017, from www.whfoods.com/genpage.php?tname=foodspice&dbid=58.

Gillette-Guyonnet, S., Secher, M., Vellas, B. (2013). Nutrition and neurodegeneration: epidemiological evidence and challenges for future research. *British Journal of Clinical Pharmacology, 75*(3), 738–755.

Gillette-Guyonnet, S., Vellas, B. (2008). Caloric restriction and brain function. *Current Opinion in Clinical Nutrition and Metabolic Care, 11,* 686–692.

Ginger. (n.d.). Retrieved January 11, 2017, from www.whfoods.com /genpage.php?tname=foodspice&dbid=72.

Greger, M., M.D. (2015, January 26). NutritionFacts.org. Retrieved January 12, 2017, from http://nutritionfacts.org/topics/flax-seeds/.

Guan, J. Z., Guan, W. P., Maeda, T., Makino, N. (2011). Effect of vitamin E administration on the elevated oxygen stress and the telomeric and subtelomeric status in Alzheimer's disease. *Gerontology, 58*(1), 62–69.

Harrison, F. E. (2012). A critical review of vitamin C for the prevention of age-related cognitive decline and Alzheimer's disease. *Journal of Alzheimer's Disease, 29*(4), 711–726.

Health benefits of millet (a gluten-free grain from India). Retrieved January 11, 2017, from www.healwithfood.org/health-benefits /millet-grain-gluten-free.php.

Health food trends—beans and legumes. (n.d.). Retrieved March 9, 2017, from medlineplus.gov/ency/patientinstructions/000726.htm.

Health properties of tomatoes. (n.d.). Retrieved January 10, 2017, from www.webmd.com/food-recipes/features/health-properties-tomatoes#1.

Hebert, L. E., Weuve, J., Scherr, P. A., Evans, D. A. (2013). Alzheimer disease in the United States (2010–2050) estimated using the 2010 census. *Neurology, 80,* 1778–1783.

Henderson, S. T., Vogel, J. L., Barr, L. J., Garvin, F., Jones, J. J., Costantini, L. C. (2009). Study of the ketogenic agent AC-1202 in mild to moderate Alzheimer's disease: a randomized, double-blind, placebo-controlled, multicenter trial. *Nutrition & Metabolism (London) 6,* 31.

Heude, B., Ducimetière, P., Berr, C. (2003). Cognitive decline and fatty acid composition of erythrocyte membranes—the EVA Study. *American Journal of Clinical Nutrition, 77,* 803–808.

Ho, L., Chen, L. H., Wang, J., Zhao, W., Talcott, S. T., Ono, K. . . . Pasinetti, G. M. (2009). Heterogeneity in red wine polyphenolic contents differentially influences Alzheimer's disease-type neuropathology and cognitive deterioration. *Journal of Alzheimer's Disease, 16*(1), 59–72.

Hotting, K., Roder, B. (2013). Beneficial effects of physical exercise on neuroplasticity and cognition. *Neuroscience & Biobehavioral Reviews, 9,* 2243–2257.

How citrus fruit helps with Alzheimer's prevention. (2016, September 5). Retrieved January 11, 2017, from http://theadplan.com/alzheimersdietblog/alzheimers-prevention-2/how-citrus-fruit-helps-with-alzheimers-prevention/.

How vitamin K is good for the brain and Alzheimer's prevention. (2016, August 16). Retrieved January 10, 2017, from www.alzheimers.net/2014-07-09/vitamin-k-alzheimers-prevention/.

Hu, N., Yu, J. T., Tan, L., Wang, Y. L., Sun, L., Tan, L. (2013). Nutrition and the risk of Alzheimer's disease. *Biomed Research International,* 524820.

The impact of supplemental macular carotenoids in Alzheimer's disease: a randomized clinical trial. (n.d.). Retrieved January 10, 2017, from www.ncbi.nlm.nih.gov/pubmed/25408222.

Inflammation in Alzheimer's disease: relevance to pathogenesis and therapy. (2010). Retrieved January 10, 2017, from www.ncbi.nlm.nih.gov/pmc/articles/PMC2874260/.

Is sleep a modifiable risk factor for Alzheimer's disease? (2015). Retrieved March 9, 2017, from www.asaging.org/blog /sleep-modifiable-risk-factor-alzheimers-disease.

Isaacson, R. S., Ochner, C. N. (2016). *The Alzheimer's prevention & treatment diet: using nutrition to combat the effects of Alzheimer's disease.* Garden City Park, NY: Square One Publishers, Inc.

Jicha, G. A., Carr, S. A. (2010). Conceptual evolution in Alzheimer's disease: implications for understanding the clinical phenotype of progressive neurodegenerative disease. *Journal of Alzheimer's Disease, 19,* 253–272.

Jicha, G. A., Markesbery, W. R. (2010). Omega-3 fatty acids: potential role in the management of early Alzheimer's disease. *Journal of Clinical Interventions in Aging, 5,* 45–61.

Jimenez-Jimenez, F. J., Molina, J. A., de Bustos, F., Orti-Pareja, M., Benito-Leon, J., Tallon-Barranco, A. . . . Arenas, J. (1999). Serum levels of beta-carotene, alpha-carotene and vitamin A in patients with Alzheimer's disease. *European Journal of Neurology, 6*(4), 495–497.

Jones, Q. R., Warford, J., Rupasinghe, H. P., Robertson, G. S. (2012). Target-based selection of flavonoids for neurodegenerative disorders. *Trends in Pharmacological Sciences, 33*(11), 602-610.

Kamphuis, P. J., Scheltens, P. (2010). Can nutrients prevent or delay onset of Alzheimer's disease? *Journal of Alzheimer's Disease, 20,* 765–775.

Kamphuis, P. J., Verhey, F. R., Olde Rikkert, M. G., Twisk, J. W., Swinkels, S. H., Scheltens, P. (2011). Efficacy of a medical food on cognition in Alzheimer's disease: results from secondary analyses of a randomized, controlled trial. *The Journal of Nutrition Health and Aging, 15,* 720–724.

Kaneai, N., Arai, M., Takatsu, H., Fukui, K., Urano, S. (2012). Vitamin E inhibits oxidative stress-induced denaturation of nerve terminal proteins involved in neurotransmission. *Journal of Alzheimer's Disease, 28*(1), 183–189.

Kang, J. H., Ascherio, A., Grodstein, F. (2005). Fruit and vegetable consumption and cognitive decline in aging women. *Annals of Neurology, 57,* 713–720.

Kashiwaya, Y., Bergman, C., Lee, J. H., Wan, R., King, M. T., Mughal, M. R. . . . Veech, R. L. (2013). A ketone ester diet exhibits anxiolytic and cognition-sparing properties, and lessens amyloid and tau pathologies in a mouse model of Alzheimer's disease. *Neurobiology of Aging, 34,* 1530 1539.

Katz, R., Edelson, M. (2015). *The healthy mind cookbook.* Berkeley, CA: Ten Speed Press.

Kent, K., Charlton, K., Roodenrys, S., Batterham, M., Potter, J., Traynor, V. . . . Richards, R. (2015). Consumption of anthocyanin-rich cherry juice for 12 weeks improves memory and cognition in older adults with mild-to-moderate dementia. *European Journal of Nutrition, 56*(1):333-341.

Khanna, S., Parinandi, N. L., Kotha, S. R., Roy, S., Rink, C., Bibus, D., Sen, C. K. (2010). Nanomolar vitamin E α-tocotrienol inhibits glutamate-induced activation of phospholipase A2 and causes neuroprotection. *Journal of Neurochemistry, 112*(5), 1249–1260.

Knopman, D. S., DeKosky, S. T., Cummings, J. L., Chui, H., Corey-Bloom, J., Relkin N., Stevens, J. C. (2001). Practice parameter: diagnosis of dementia (an evidence-based review). Report of the Quality Standards Subcommittee of the American Academy of Neurology. *Neurology, 56,* 1143–1153.

Kryscio, R. J., Abner, E. L., Schmitt, F. A., Goodman, P. J., Mendiondo, M., Caban-Holt, A. . . . Crowley, J. J. (2013). A randomized controlled Alzheimer's disease prevention trial's evolution into an exposure trial: the PREADViSE trial. *The Journal of Nutrition Health and Aging, 17,* 72–75.

Laitinen, M. H., Ngandu, T., Rovio, S., Helkala, E. L., Uusitalo, U., Viitanen, M. . . . Kivipelto, M. (2006). Fat intake at midlife and risk of dementia and Alzheimer's disease: a population-based study. *Dementia and Geriatric Cognitive Disorders, 22,* 99–107.

Lau, F. C., Shukitt-Hale, B., Joseph, J. A. (2007). Nutritional intervention in brain aging: reducing the effects of inflammation and oxidative stress. *Sub-cellular Biochemistry, 42,* 299–318.

Lee, J. G., Yon, J. M., Lin, C., Jung, A.Y., Jung, K.Y., Nam, S. Y. (2012). Combined treatment with capsaicin and resveratrol enhances neuroprotection against glutamate-induced toxicity in mouse cerebral cortical neurons. *Food Chemical Toxicology, 50*(11), 3877–3885.

Lemon/limes. (n.d.). Retrieved January 11, 2017, from www.whfoods.com /genpage.php?tname=foodspice&dbid=27.

Lopes da Silva, S., Vellas, B., Elemans, S., Luchsinger, J., Kamphuis, P., Yaffe, K. . . . Stijnen, T. (2014). Plasma nutrient status of patients with Alzheimer's disease: systematic review and meta-analysis. *Alzheimer's & Dementia, 10,* 485–502.

Luchsinger, J. A., Tang, M. X., Shea, S., Mayeux, R. (2002). Caloric intake and the risk of Alzheimer's disease. *Archives of Neurology, 59,* 1258–1263.

Malaguarnera, M., Ferri, R., Bella, R., Alagona, G., Carnemolla, A., Pennisi, G. (2004). Homocysteine, vitamin B_{12} and folate in vascular dementia and in Alzheimer disease. *Clinical Chemistry and Laboratory Medicine, 42,* 1032–1035.

Mango fruit nutrition facts and health benefits. (n.d.). Retrieved January 11, 2017, from www.nutrition-and-you.com/mango-fruit.html.

Martínez-Lapiscina, E. H., Clavero, P., Toledo, E., Estruch, R., Salas-Salvado, J., San Julian, B. . . . Martinez-Gonzalez, M. A. (2013). Mediterranean diet improves cognition: the PREDIMED-NAVARRA randomized trial. *Journal of Neurology, Neurosurgery and Psychiatry, 84*(12), 1318–25.

Masse, I., Bordet, R., Deplanque, D., Al Khedr, A., Richard, F., Libersa, C. . . . Pasquier, F. (2005). Lipid lowering agents are associated with a slower cognitive decline in Alzheimer's disease. *Journal of Neurology, Neurosurgery and Psychiatry, 76,* 1624–1629.

Mateljan, G. (2015). *The world's healthiest foods* (2nd ed.). New York: GMF Publishing.

Mayer, E. A., Knight, R., Mazmanian, J. F., Cryan, J. F., Tillisch, K. (2014). Gut microbes and the brain: paradigm shift in neuroscience. *Neuroscience, 34*(46), 15490–15496.

Medium chain triglycerides. (2016, April 28). Retrieved January 12, 2017, from www.alzdiscovery.org/cognitive-vitality/ratings /medium-chain-triglycerides.

Mielke, M. M., Prashanthi, V., Rocca, W. A. (2014). Clinical epidemiology of Alzheimer's disease: assessing sex and gender differences. *Clinical Epidemiology, 6,* 37–48.

Miller, E. R. III, Pastor-Barriuso, R., Dalal, D., Riemersma, R. A., Appel, L. J., Guallar, E. (2005). Meta-analysis: high-dosage vitamin E supplementation may increase all-cause mortality. *Annals of Internal Medicine, 142,* 37–46.

Millet. (n.d.). Retrieved January 11, 2017, from www.whfoods.com /genpage.php?tname=foodspice&dbid=53.

Monti, M. C., Margarucci, L., Tosco, A., Riccio, R., Casapullo, A. (2011). New insights on the interaction mechanism between tau protein and oleocanthal, an extra-virgin olive-oil bioactive component. *Food & Function, 2,* 423–428.

Morris, M. C., Evans, D. A., Tangney, C. C., Bienias, J. L., Schneider, J. A., Wilson, R. S., Scherr, P. A. (2006). Dietary copper and high saturated and trans fat intakes associated with cognitive decline. *Archives of Neurology, 63,* 1085–1088.

Morris, M. C., Evans, D. A., Tangney, C. C., Bienias, J. L., Wilson, R. S. (2006). Associations of vegetable and fruit consumption with age-related cognitive change. *Neurology, 67,* 1370–1376.

Morris, M. C., Evans, D. A., Tangney, C. C., Bienias, J. L., Wilson, R. S., Aggarwal, N. T., Scherr, P. A. (2005). Relation of the tocopherol forms to incident Alzheimer disease and cognitive change. *American Journal of Clinical Nutrition, 81,* 508–514.

Morris, M. C., Tangney, C. C. (2014). Dietary fat composition and dementia risk. *Neurobiology of Aging, 35*(2), S59–S64.

Morris, M. D., Schneider, J. A., Tangney. (2006). Thoughts on B-vitamins and dementia. *Journal of Alzheimers Disease, 9*(4); 429–433.

Morris, M. S. (2002). Folate, homocysteine, and neurological function. *Nutrition in Clinical Care, 5*(3), 124–132.

Morris, M. S. (2003). Homocysteine and Alzheimer's disease. *The Lancet Neurology, 2,* 425–428.

Morris, M. S. (2012). The role of B vitamins in preventing and treating cognitive impairment and decline. *Advances in Nutrition, 3,* 801–812.

Mythri, R. B., Bharath, M. M. (2012). Curcumin: a potential neuroprotective agent in Parkinson's disease. *Current Pharmaceutical Design, 18*(1), 91–99.

Napa Cabbage. (2015, January 23). Retrieved January 10, 2017, from awomanshealth.com/napa-cabbage/.

Neal, B. N. (2014). Dietary and lifestyle guidelines for the prevention of Alzheimer's disease. *Neurobiology of Aging, 35,* S74–S78.

Nishida, Y., Yokota, T., Takahashi, T., Uchihara, T., Jishage, K., Mizusawa, H. (2006). Deletion of vitamin E enhances phenotype of Alzheimer disease model mouse. *Biochemical and Biophysical Research Communications, 350,* 530–536.

Nutmeg nutrition facts, medicinal properties and health benefits. (n.d.). Retrieved January 11, 2017, from www.nutrition-and-you.com /nutmeg.html.

Nutrition. (n.d.). Retrieved January 11, 2017, from www.californiaavocado .com/nutrition.

Nutrition and prevention of Alzheimer's dementia. (2014). Retrieved January 10, 2017, from www.ncbi.nlm.nih.gov/pmc/articles /PMC4202787/.

Obrenovich, M. E., Nair, N. G., Beyaz, A., Aliev, G., Reddy, V. P. (2010). The role of polyphenolic antioxidants in health, disease, and aging. *Rejuvenation Research, 13*(6), 631–643.

Okereke, O. I., Rosner, B. A., Kim, D. H., Kang, J. H., Cook, N. R., Manson, J. E., . . . Grodstein, F. (2012). Dietary fat types and 4-year cognitive change in community-dwelling older women. *Annals of Neurology, 72,* 124–134.

Olive oil, extra virgin. (n.d.). Retrieved January 13, 2017, from www.whfoods.com/genpage.php?tname=foodspice&dbid=132.

Olive oil: health benefits, nutritional information. (2016). Retrieved March 9, 2017, from www.medicalnewstoday.com /articles/266258.php.

Panza, F., Frisardi, V., Capurso, C., Imbimbo, B. P., Vendemiale, G., Santamato, A., Solfrizzi, V. (2010). Metabolic syndrome and cognitive impairment: current epidemiology and possible underlying mechanisms. *Journal of Alzheimer's Disease, 21,* 691–724.

Parsley nutrition facts and health benefits. (n.d.). Retrieved January 11, 2017, from www.nutrition-and-you.com/parsley.html.

Pasinetti, G. M., Eberstein, J. A. (2008). Metabolic syndrome and the role of dietary lifestyles in Alzheimer's disease. *Journal of Neurochemistry, 106,* 1503–14.

Pervaiz, S., Holme, A. L. (2009). Resveratrol: its biologic targets and functional activity. *Antioxidants & Redox Signaling, 11,* 2851–2897.

Plantains nutrition facts and health benefits. (n.d.). Retrieved January 11, 2017, from www.nutrition-and-you.com/plantains.html.

Pocernich, C. B., Lange, M. L., Sultana, R., Butterfield, D. A. (2011). Nutritional approaches to modulate oxidative stress in Alzheimer's disease. *Current Alzheimer Research, 8,* 452–469.

Presse, N., Belleville, S., Gaudreau, P., Greenwood, C. E., Kergoat, M. J., Morais, J. A. . . . Ferland, G. (2013). Vitamin K status and cognitive function in healthy older adults, *Neurobiology of Aging, 34*(12), 2777–2783.

Quinn, J. F., Raman, R., Thomas, R. G., Yurko-Mauro, K., Nelson, E. B., Van Dyck, C. . . . Aisen, P. S. (2010). Docosahexaenoic acid supplementation and cognitive decline in Alzheimer disease: a randomized trial. *Journal of the American Medical Assocation, 304,* 1903–1911.

Rafii, M. S., Walsh, S., Little, J. T., Behan, K., Reynolds, B., Ward, C. . . . Aisen, P. S. (2011). A phase II trial of huperzine A in mild to moderate Alzheimer disease. *Neurology, 76,* 1389–1394.

Ranking seafood: which fish are most nutritious? (n.d.). Retrieved March 9, 2017, from www.askdrsears.com/topics/feeding-eating /family-nutrition/fish/ranking-seafood-which-fish-are -most-nutritious.

Rao, A. V., Balachandran, B. (2002). Role of oxidative stress and antioxidants in neurodegenerative diseases. *Nutritional Neuroscience, 5,* 291–309.

Reger, M. A., Henderson, S. T., Hale, C., Cholerton, B., Baker, L. D., Watson, G. S. . . . Craft, S. (2004). Effects of beta-hydroxybutyrate on cognition in memory-impaired adults. *Neurobiology of Aging, 25,* 311–314.

Reynolds, E. H. (2002, June 22). Folic acid, ageing, depression, and dementia. Retrieved January 10, 2017, from www.ncbi.nlm.nih.gov /pmc/articles/PMC1123448/.

Ringman, J. M., Frautschy, S. A., Teng, E., Begum, A. N., Bardens, J., Beigi, M. . . . Cole, G. M. (2008). Oral curcumin for the treatment of mild-to-moderate Alzheimer's disease: tolerability and clinical and biomarker efficacy results of a placebo-controlled 24-week study. *Proceedings of the International Conference on Alzheimer's Disease.* Chicago, IL.

Rockwood, K. (2006). Epidemiological and clinical trials evidence about a preventive role for statins in Alzheimer's disease. *Acta Neurologica Scandinavica Supplement, 185,* 71–77.

Role of thiamine in Alzheimer's disease. (2011, December 26). Retrieved January 12, 2017, from www.ncbi.nlm.nih.gov/pubmed/22218733.

Rubio-Perez, J. M., Morillas-Ruiz, J. M. (2012). A review: inflammatory process in Alzheimer's disease, role of cytokines. *The Scientific World Journal, 756357,* 1–15.

Sailors' scurvy before and after James Lind—a reassessment. (n.d.). Retrieved January 11, 2017, from www.ncbi.nlm.nih.gov /pubmed/19519673.

Sangiorgio, M. (2016, August 11). Black currant: a natural tool to fight Alzheimer's. Retrieved January 11, 2017, from www.senioroutlooktoday.com/black-currant-a-natural -tool-to-fight-alzheimers/.

Sano, M., Bell, K. L., Galasko, D., Galvin, J. E., Thomas, R. G., van Dyck, C. H., Aisen, P. S. (2011). A randomized, double-blind, placebo-controlled trial of simvastatin to treat Alzheimer disease. *Neurology, 77,* 556–563.

Sano, M., Ernesto, C., Thomas, R. G., Klauber, M. R., Schafer, K., Grundman, M. . . . Thal, L. G. (1997). A controlled trial of selegiline, α-tocopherol, or both as treatment for Alzheimer's disease. The Alzheimer's Disease Cooperative Study. *New England Journal of Medicine, 336,* 1216–1222.

Saturated fat, regardless of type, linked with increased heart disease risk. (2016). Retrieved January 10, 2017, from www.hsph.harvard.edu /nutritionsource/2016/12/19/saturated-fat-regardless-of-type -found-linked-with-increased-heart-disease-risk/.

Scarmeas, N., Luchsinger, J. A., Mayeux, R., Stern, Y. (2007). Mediterranean diet and Alzheimer disease mortality. *Neurology, 69,* 1084–1093.

Scarmeas, N., Stern, Y., Tang, M. X., Mayeux, R., Luchsinger, J. A. (2006). Mediterranean diet and risk for Alzheimer's disease. *Annals of Neurology, 59,* 912–921.

Schrag, M., Mueller, C., Zabel, M., Crofton, A., Kirsch, W. M., Ghribi, O. . . . Perry, G. (2013). Oxidative stress in blood in Alzheimer's disease and mild cognitive impairment: a meta-analysis. *Neurobiology of Disease, 59,* 100–110.

The search for Alzheimer's prevention strategies. (2016). Retrieved January 10, 2017, from www.nia.nih.gov/alzheimers/publication /preventing-alzheimers-disease/search-alzheimers-prevention -strategies.

Seshadri, S., Beiser, A., Selhub, J., Jacques, P. F., Rosenberg, I. H., D'Agostino, R. B. . . . Wolf, P. A. (2002). Plasma homocysteine as a risk factor for dementia and Alzheimer's disease. *New England Journal of Medicine, 346,* 476–483.

Shah, R. (2013). The role of nutrition and diet in Alzheimer disease: a systematic review. *Journal of the American Medical Directors Association, 14,* 398–402.

Shah, R. C., Kamphuis, P. J., Leurgans, S., Swinkels, S. H., Sadowsky, C. H., Bongers, A. . . . Bennett, D. A. (2013). The S-Connect study: results from a randomized, controlled trial of Souvenaid in mild-to-moderate Alzheimer's disease. *Alzheimers Research & Therapy, 5,* 59.

Smith, A. D., Smith, S. M., de Jager, C. A., Whitbread, P., Johnston, C., Agacinski, G. . . . Refsum, H. (2010). Homocysteine-lowering by B vitamins slows the rate of accelerated brain atrophy in mild cognitive impairment: a randomized controlled trial. PLOS ONE, 5, e12244.

Smith, M. A., Zhu, X., Tabaton, M., Liu, G., McKeel, D. W. Jr., Cohen, M. L. . . . Perry, G. (2010). Increased iron and free radical generation in preclinical Alzheimer disease and mild cognitive impairment. *Journal of Alzheimer's Disease, 19*(1), 353–372.

Snitz, B. E., O'Meara, E. S., Carlson, M. C., Arnold, A. M., Ives, D. G., Rapp, S. R. . . . DeKosky, S. T. (2009). Ginkgo biloba for preventing cognitive decline in older adults: a randomized trial. *Journal of the American Medical Association, 302,* 2663–2670.

Sofi, F., Macchi, C., Abbate, R., Gensini, G. F., Casini, A. (2010). Effectiveness of the Mediterranean diet: can it help delay or prevent Alzheimer's disease? *Journal of Alzheimer's Disease, 20,* 795–801.

Solfrizzi, V., Panza, F., Frisardi, V., Seripa, D., Logroscino ,G., Imbimbo, B. P. . . . Pilotto, A. (2011). Diet and Alzheimer's disease risk factors or prevention: the current evidence. *Expert Review of Neurotherapeutics, 11,* 677–708.

Solfrizzi, V., Scafato, E., Capurso, C., D'Introno, A., Colacicco, A. M., Frisardi, V. . . . Panza, F. (2010). Metabolic syndrome and the risk of vascular dementia: the Italian Longitudinal Study on Ageing. *Journal of Neurology, Neurosurgery and Psychiatry, 81,* 433–440.

Spencer, J. P. (2009). Flavonoids and brain health: multiple effects underpinned by common mechanisms. *Genes & Nutrition, 4*(4), 243–250.

Stern, Y. (2012). Cognitive reserve in ageing and Alzheimer's disease. *The Lancet Neurology, 11,* 1006–1012.

Sulforaphane as a potential protective phytochemical against neurodegenerative diseases. (2013). Retrieved January 10, 2017, from http://theconversation.com/what-can-beagles-teach-us-about-alzheimers-disease-35588.

Swaminathan, A., Jicha, G. A. (2014). Nutrition and prevention of Alzheimer's dementia. *Frontiers in Aging Neuroscience, 6,* 282.

Szalay, J. (2016, April 25). Cauliflower: health benefits and nutrition facts. Retrieved January 5, 2016, from www.livescience.com /54552-cauliflower-nutrition.html.

Tara Gidus, MS, RD, CSSD, LD/N. (2012, February 22). (n.d.). Super food of the week: health benefits of plantains. Retrieved January 11, 2017, from www.healthline.com/health-blogs/diet-diva /health-benefits-plantains.

Thaipisuttikul, P., Galvin, J. E. (2012). Use of medical foods and nutritional approaches in the treatment of Alzheimer's disease. *Clinical Practice (London) 9*, 199–209.

Tucker, A. M., Stern, Y. (2011). Cognitive reserve in aging. *Current Alzheimer Research, 8*, 354–360.

Tworoger, S. S., Lee, S., Schernhammer, E. S., Grodstein, F. (2006). The association of self-reported sleep duration, difficulty sleeping, and snoring with cognitive function in older women. *Alzheimer Disease and Associated Disorders, 20*, 41–48.

University of Illinois Extension. (n.d.). Pumpkin nutrition. Retrieved January 12, 2017, from https://extension.illinois.edu/pumpkins /nutrition.cfm.

Vogel, T., Dali-Youcef, N., Kaltenbach, G., Andrès, E. (2009). Homocysteine, vitamin B_{12}, folate and cognitive functions: a systematic and critical review of the literature. *International Journal of Clinical Practice, 63*, 1061–1067.

Wang, Y., Yin, H., Wang, L., Shuboy, A., Lou, J., Han, B. . . . Li, J. (2013). Curcumin as a potential treatment for Alzheimer's disease: a study of the effects of curcumin on hippocampal expression of glial fibrillary acidic protein. *American Journal of Chinese Medicine, 41*, 59–70.

Ware, Megan. (2015, September 29). Cauliflower: health benefits, nutritional information. Retrieved January 10, 2017, from www .medicalnewstoday.com/articles/282844.php.

Ware, Megan. (2016, September 14). Chickpeas: health benefits, nutritional information. Retrieved January 11, 2017, from www.medicalnewstoday .com/articles/280244.php.

Ware, Megan. (2016, January 5). Ginger: health benefits, facts, research. Retrieved January 11, 2017, from www.medicalnewstoday.com /articles/265990.php.

Ware, Megan. (2015, October 21). Mangoes: health benefits, nutritional breakdown. Retrieved January 11, 2017, from www.medicalnewstoday .com/articles/275921.php.

Ware, Megan. (2016, February 16). Mint: health benefits, uses and risks. Retrieved January 11, 2017, from www.medicalnewstoday.com /articles/275944.php.

Ware, Megan. (2016, October 20). Watercress: health benefits and nutritional breakdown. Retrieved January 11, 2017, from www .medicalnewstoday.com/articles/285412.php.

Watercress nutrition facts. (n.d.). Retrieved March 9, 2017, from www.nutrition-and-you.com/watercress.html.

Weih, M., Wiltfang, J., Kornhuber, J. (2007). Non-pharmacologic prevention of Alzheimer's disease: nutritional and life-style risk factors. *Journal of Neural Transmission, 114,* 1187–1197.

What is black currant good for? (n.d.). Retrieved January 11, 2017, from http://foodfacts.mercola.com/black-currant.html.

What is your risk?—heredity and late-onset Alzheimer's disease. (2016). Retrieved January 10, 2017, from www.brightfocus.org/alzheimers /article/what-your-risk-heredity-and-late-onset-alzheimers-disease.

Wheeler, M. (2013, August 20). UCLA study suggests iron is at core of Alzheimer's disease. Retrieved January 11, 2017, from newsroom.ucla.edu/releases/ucla-study-suggests-that-iron-247864.

Williams, R. J., Spencer, J. P. (2012). Flavonoids, cognition, and dementia: actions, mechanisms, and potential therapeutic utility for Alzheimer disease. *Free Radical Biology and Medicine, 52*(1), 35–45.

Yaffe, K., Laffan, A. M., Harrison, S. L., Redline, S., Spira, A. P., Ensrud, K. E. . . . Stone, K. L. (2011). Sleep-disordered breathing, hypoxia, and risk of mild cognitive impairment and dementia in older women. *Journal of the American Medical Association, 306*, 613–619.

Yang, X., Dai, G., Li, G., Yang, E. S. (2010). Coenzyme Q10 reduces beta-amyloid plaque in an APP/PS1 transgenic mouse model of Alzheimer's disease. *Journal of Molecular Neuroscience, 41*, 110–113.

Yatin, S. M., Varadarajan, S., Butterfield, D. A. (2000). Vitamin E prevents Alzheimer's amyloid β-peptide (1-42)-induced neuronal protein oxidation and reactive oxygen species production. *Journal of Alzheimer's Disease, 2*(2), 123–131.

Yehuda, S., Rabinovitz, S., Mostofsky, D. I. (2005). Essential fatty acids and the brain: from infancy to aging. *Neurobiology of Aging, 26* (Supplement 1), 98–102.

Yurko-Mauro, K., McCarthy, D., Rom, D., Nelson, E. B., Ryan, A. S., Blackwell, A. . . . Stedman, M. (2010). Beneficial effects of docosahexaenoic acid on cognition in age-related cognitive decline. *Alzheimers Dementia, 6*, 456 464.

Zandi, P. P., Anthony, J. C., Khachaturian, A. S, Stone, S. V., Gustafson, D., Tschanz, J. T. . . . Breitner, J. C. (2004). Reduced risk of Alzheimer disease in users of antioxidant vitamin supplements: the Cache County Study. *Archives of Neurology, 61*(1), 82–88.

Zhang, J., Cao, Q., Li, S., Lu, X., Zhao, Y., Guan, J. S. . . . Chen, G. Q. (2013). 3-Hydroxybutyrate methyl ester as a potential drug against Alzheimer's disease via mitochondria protection mechanism. *Biomaterials, 34*, 7552–7562.

Zhang, S., Rocourt, C., Cheng, W. H. (2010). Selenoproteins and the aging brain. *Mechanisms of Ageing and Development, 131,* 253–260.

Zilberter, M., Ivanov, A., Ziyatdinova, S., Mukhtarov, M., Malkov, A., Alpár, A., Zilberter, Y. (2013). Dietary energy substrates reverse early neuronal hyperactivity in a mouse model of Alzheimer's disease. *Journal of Neurochemistry, 125,* 157–171.

The Dirty Dozen & the Clean Fifteen

A nonprofit environmental watchdog organization called Environmental Working Group (EWG) looks at data supplied by the US Department of Agriculture (USDA) and the Food and Drug Administration (FDA) about pesticide residues. Each year it compiles a list of the best and worst pesticide loads found in commercial crops. You can use these lists to decide which fruits and vegetables to buy organic to minimize your exposure to pesticides and which produce is considered safe enough to buy conventionally. This does not mean they are pesticide-free, though, so wash these fruits and vegetables thoroughly.

These lists change every year, so make sure you look up the most recent one before you fill your shopping cart. You'll find the most recent lists as well as a guide to pesticides in produce at EWG.org /FoodNews.

2017 Dirty Dozen

Apples
Celery
Cherries
Grapes
Nectarines
Peaches
Pears
Potatoes
Spinach
Strawberries
Sweet bell peppers
Tomatoes

In addition to the Dirty Dozen, the EWG added one type of produce contaminated with highly toxic organophosphate insecticides:

Hot peppers

2017 Clean Fifteen

Asparagus
Avocados
Cabbage
Cantaloupes (domestic)
Cauliflower
Eggplants
Grapefruits
Honeydew melons
Kiwis
Mangos
Onions
Papayas*
Pineapples
Sweet corn*
Sweet peas (frozen)

A small amount of sweet corn and papaya sold in the United States is produced from genetically modified seeds. Buy organic varieties of these crops if you want to avoid genetically modified produce.

Measurement Conversions

Volume Equivalents (Liquid)

US STANDARD	US STANDARD (OUNCES)	METRIC (APPROXIMATE)
2 tablespoons	1 fl. oz.	30 mL
¼ cup	2 fl. oz.	60 mL
½ cup	4 fl. oz.	120 mL
1 cup	8 fl. oz.	240 mL
1½ cups	12 fl. oz.	355 mL
2 cups or 1 pint	16 fl. oz.	475 mL
4 cups or 1 quart	32 fl. oz.	1 L
1 gallon	128 fl. oz.	4 L

Oven Temperatures

FAHRENHEIT (F)	CELSIUS (C) (APPROXIMATE)
250°F	120°C
300°F	150°C
325°F	165°C
350°F	180°C
375°F	190°C
400°F	200°C
425°F	220°C
450°F	230°C

Volume Equivalents (Dry)

US STANDARD	METRIC (APPROXIMATE)
⅛ teaspoon	0.5 mL
¼ teaspoon	1 mL
½ teaspoon	2 mL
¾ teaspoon	4 mL
1 teaspoon	5 mL
1 tablespoon	15 mL
¼ cup	59 mL
⅓ cup	79 mL
½ cup	118 mL
⅔ cup	156 mL
¾ cup	177 mL
1 cup	235 mL
2 cups or 1 pint	475 mL
3 cups	700 mL
4 cups or 1 quart	1 L

Weight Equivalents

US STANDARD	METRIC (APPROXIMATE)
½ ounce	15 g
1 ounce	30 g
2 ounces	60 g
4 ounces	115 g
8 ounces	225 g
12 ounces	340 g
16 ounces or 1 pound	455 g

Index

C

V

Vegetables, 30, 59–69
Vitamins, 14

W

Wake Forest School of Medicine, 7
Walnuts, 85, 87
Wasabi, 53
Watercress, 58
Weight, 105
Western diet, 15

Wheat germ, 82

Wheat germ, 82
Whole grains, 32, 79–82
Winter squash, 68

Y

Yams, 69
Yogurt, 94

Z

Zucchini, 69

Acknowledgments

We would like to acknowledge and express sincere thanks to our families and friends for enduring the months of neglect while we worked on this publication.

To Sue's loving husband, Rod, who picked up the slack around the house, was endlessly patient, and was the best cheerleader, stress reducer and friend throughout the process. To daughters, Sarah and Sena, the sweetest and most supportive girls in the world. Thanks for even making dinner a few times! To Sue's forever-friend and business partner, Maureen Sykes, for holding up both ends of the partnership while this project was in full swing.

To SeAnne's children, Siraj, Signey, and Seagen, who have provided support and encouragement in the balance between motherhood and professionalism. To her wonderful husband, John, who is a great mentor, partner, friend, and exercise buddy.

To our parents—our biggest fans and role models—thank you! Without our beautiful moms, the passion behind this book would not have been the same. We miss them every day.

We are extraordinarily grateful to the bright college students who sacrificed their time to contribute to this endeavor. Elizabeth "Libby" Reynolds, you will be an amazing registered dietitian one day! Sarah Stillman, your linguistics and sharp editing skills have finally exceeded those of your mother. We can't wait to see how far you'll go in this world.

To our biggest supporters: Jamie Talan, our local neurology buff, mentor, and friend; Maria Ortega, marketing and communications manager from the University of Idaho; and all of the hardworking and loyal Registered Dietitian Nutritionists from the Idaho Academy of Nutrition and Dietetics and our other professional networks—thanks! Without all of you, we would be nowhere.

And last but not least, we would like to thank our amazing team at Callisto Media, including our editor Stacy Wagner-Kinnear. To the countless others who have helped and supported this book behind the scenes, you do exemplary work and we salute you!

About the Authors

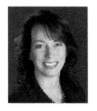

Sue Stillman Linja, RDN, LD, is cofounder, with SeAnne Safaii-Waite, of Nutrition and Wellness Associates. Sue is also president of S&S Nutrition Network, as well as cofounder and vice president of LTC Nutrition Counseling. Having worked in geriatrics for the entirety of her career, Sue is passionate about helping others age healthfully. Her main focus is on working with long-term care facilities in a variety of capacities, including nutrition services director, clinical dietitian, health facility surveyor, and dietitian consultant. Sue lives with her husband and children in Idaho.

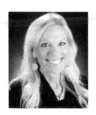

SeAnne Safaii-Waite, PhD, RDN, LD, is Associate Professor of Nutrition and Dietetics at the University of Idaho. With Sue Stillman Linja, she is cofounder of Nutrition and Wellness Associates. SeAnne is a registered dietitian, nutrition communications professional, and educator. The author of many journal articles and textbook chapters, SeAnne is also a sought-after nutrition expert for websites, newspapers, and local television networks. She is a recipient of the Academy of Nutrition and Dietetics' Outstanding Dietitian Award. SeAnne and her husband live in Idaho.

Printed in the USA
FMT401.142506281017

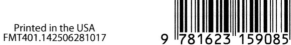